Get Fit, Stay Fit, Remain Fit

Create Habits that Last

Glen Gosch

Cover design and layout by Megan Raburn

ISBN: 0615770932
ISBN-13: 978-0615770932

DEDICATION

For my best friend and wife Jaki. Your encouragement and smile keep me going. You are my first editor of every book or project that I dream up and I am grateful for all of your help. Thank you for being by my side as I chase my dreams.

CONTENTS

A NOTE FROM THE INDIE AUTHOR/PUBLISHER/EDITOR

Hi, my name is Glen Gosch, you can call me Glen. Get Fit Stay Fit Remain Fit is a piece written, published, and edited by me. I feel blessed to live in a time where a person with a vision can put his thoughts and words to paper (or digital format) the way he pleases. In this first print addition I chose the DIY model. I thought about going the query, agent, publisher route, hoping someone gives this book a blessing, but I ultimately chose to just do it. I went through the 'What if their are speling mistakes, grammar, issues, format issues, etc.?" thoughts in my head, and ultimately I decided to rely on my own knowledge and experience, and carefully comb the book for errors with a little help from my friends. I don't think there are any errors as bad as the previous sentence. That said, to this day I am still surprised at some of the mistakes that I catch in best-selling books from major publishers. I've seen words left out, misspelled words, grammar errors, and more in even some of the more popular titles of our time. So as you read this book I make no apologies for uncaught mistakes – I'm playing the Human Card. If the big boys can make mistakes, so can I. I hope you find the book valuable, and if you can read it and walk away with something that improves your life, then I will feel truly blessed.

Part 1: How to Do It

INTRODUCTION

Each year in January the fitness industry experiences a boom. Millions of people spend money on gym memberships, fitness DVDs, exercise equipment, and supplements enthusiastically going after their goals. Some stick with it all year and achieve their goals. Most end up losing sight of their goals and fail to accomplish the weight loss, muscle gains, or body transformation they were hoping for. Sometime in February or March people hit a slump and activity decreases. People hold on to the gym membership, they keep the exercise videos in a drawer, yet the traffic at the gym thins out and the DVDs collect dust. People hope to get back at it *someday*.

That is what this book is about: staying with a fitness routine and achieving your goals. This book is filled with information, tips, and ideas that you can apply to your life. It is a book for you if you want to achieve your goals, stay with them beyond a couple of weeks or months, and remain engaged with your fitness goals for the long-term.

Ever read a book that really inspired you? What about a book that gave you some practical life lessons that caused an internal light bulb to shine bright and show you a brighter future? I certainly have. As I looked over my library of books (both in print and in audio form) from authors such as Brian Tracy, John C. Maxwell, Zig Ziglar, Jim Rohn, and Norman Vincent Peale (to name a few), I thought about some of the important lessons I have learned from their voices. I thought about the quotes that leaped off of the pages and stuck in my mind. I thought about the times I would be listening to an audio recording and say, "Oh that was good! I need to get a pen and write that down."

If you have never heard of the names mentioned in the last paragraph, I wrote this book especially for you. If you have heard of those names and have read the works from them, you'll understand where I am coming from.

If you want to read a book on how to lose weight or get in shape, where is the first place you would look? My guess would be that you would not venture into the "self-help" section or the "business" section. You would probably look in the health/fitness section of the book store (or online search category) where you would find fitness and diet books that essentially tell you *what* to do. Eat this, do this many push-ups, exercise this many days per week. There is absolutely nothing wrong with books like that, I own several that have been very useful to me, but I think what is absent (or seriously lacking) from the fitness industry are books that create a mindset allowing for readers to stay with their goals related to health and fitness.

There are a million "what to do" tools out there in the world of health. What are "what to do" tools, you ask? They are the tools that tell us do exercises A, B, and C while eating foods X, Y, and Z to get the results we want. We do not lack the knowledge of what to do to lose weight or get in shape. It has been around for decades. What we lack is the understanding of how to stay with the "what to do" information that is out there. We need to learn the steps it takes to use the tools available to us. Use the gym membership all year, keep dust from collecting on the fitness DVDs, and prevent cob webs from forming on exercise equipment in the garage. This book is not going to tell you how many push-ups and pull-ups to do or reveal the secret of six pack abs through a particular exercise. This book is going to show you how to achieve the results you want by *changing your habits*, and not just temporarily.

The words written here are the result of my own learning from reading a lot of books, magazine articles, newsletters, and online articles. It is the result of participating in several different fitness programs, attending seminars, attending classes, and learning from some of the top trainers and coaches around. It also reflects some of my own life experiences of living a healthy lifestyle. I write from my own experience of being overweight and struggling to stay with a fitness routine, but ultimately learning how to accomplish my fitness-related goals and stay with them. I have put this all together in a concise format that provides steps you can take right away to get started on a path of achievement.

In this book we take a look at lifestyle change, goal setting, planning, tracking progress, and staying motivated with exercise. Start now and I have no doubt you will be able to live a healthy lifestyle this year, and the rest of your life. It's time to Get Fit, Stay Fit, and Remain Fit.

1. LIFESTYLE CHANGE

How do most people view the word diet? Most people view a diet as something that we do temporarily. "I'm going on a diet," for instance, is a phrase many of us use when we plan to re-shape the way we eat for a certain period of time. Another way we look at dieting is a restriction from something we are accustomed to doing. We'll take a brief break from the amount of calories, carbs, fats, or whatever the particular diet plan we set out to follow suggests. Temporary plans lead to temporary results.

When it comes to fitness there is another temporary practice that is common among us today. We see this every January as people fill up health clubs after the New Year hoping that "this year will be different." Anyone that has ever had a gym membership knows what I am talking about. January seems to be International Take Action Month in the world of fitness where New Year Resolutioners run rampant. Some continue to take action all the way to the next New Year; unfortunately most people exercise temporarily and fade out sometime in March waiting to try it again the next New Year. Temporary action leads to temporary results.

Instead of looking at physical fitness, diet, and health as something that we can fix with a temporary change in our lives, we need to focus on long-term habits and our way of life. Short-term goals, plans, and actions are a necessary part of staying with fitness activities for the entire year and the rest of your life, but they are only a part of the solution. We have to think about commitments with exercise beyond the coming weeks and months ahead.

Lotto Tickets, Jackpots, and Getting Fit Quick

We live in an instant gratification society. We like quick results. We like fast food, microwaves, drive-through windows, and instant-winner game tickets. How many people play the lottery in hopes of becoming instantly rich overnight? Millions. How many lottery winners do you personally know? My guess is zero. The same thing goes for slot machines and poker tables in Las Vegas. A small town in the middle of the desert became a large city and one of the most traveled tourist destinations in the world based off of the hope of instant success. Casino and gaming companies have become large corporations with tens of thousands of employees; all built on people's dreams of striking it rich with little or no work. How many of the current estimated 8.9 million millionaires in the United States are the recipients of winning lotto tickets and jackpots? The number is too small to even count.

When it comes to fitness we are attracted to the same type of advertising. Slim down in 6 weeks, get totally ripped in 90 days, or change your body in no time at all. While many of these programs can work and deliver great results in a quick amount of time, I have a secret for you: In order to get fit and stay fit, it is not the result of doing something for 6 weeks or 90 days – it is the result of doing something consistently over time for the long-run. There is no jackpot or winning lotto ticket when it comes to your health. To achieve results that last, we need to think about the long-term. We need to adopt a lifestyle change.

Defining Lifestyle Change

So, what exactly is a lifestyle change? According to Merriam-Webster's Dictionary, lifestyle is *the typical way of life of an individual, group, or culture*. Our habits and choices in our daily routines make up our lifestyle. In order to make this change we need to take a look at all aspects of our lives. The food we eat, the activities we participate in, the people we spend time with, the books or magazines we read, the websites that we visit – all of these things are a part of our lifestyle. Making a lifestyle change might seem like taking on a huge task; making a transformation; doing a 180 degree turn; living completely different than you do now. If you look at the big picture, it really doesn't take all that much to change. It does take some discipline. It does take some time. It does involve *some* change.

Time

There is one thing that I can assure you about the day you will have tomorrow: it will be 24 hours long. The same amount of time that I have, your neighbor has, and the same amount of time the person with the physique that you wish for has. Chances are you have several things in your day that remain constant. Most of us will sleep, eat, work, bathe, and have some other commitment to adhere to. Your day might look something like this:

Sleep	8 hours
Work	8 hours
Travel to/from work	30 minutes (at least)
Bathing/grooming	30 minutes (at least)
Time spent eating/cooking	1 hour (at least)
Further commitments	1 hour (at least)
House chores	2 hours
Total	*21 hours*

If you have 21 out of 24 hours in a day committed to certain things, you are left with about 12% of your day to do with as you please. The small decisions that you make within a small window of time during the day are what will create the lifestyle that you want, and hopefully that is a healthy and active one. Making small, little, seemingly unimportant decisions within the shortest part of your day make all the difference in the world when it comes to achieving your fitness goals.

I know that not everyone's schedule mimics the one that I used as an example, but hopefully you can see the picture that I am portraying. To make a healthy lifestyle change you do not need to change your day by 100%. You don't need to flip your entire life upside down to change your lifestyle, but you do have to change – slightly. People that exercise regularly and live an active lifestyle do not have more time during the day than anyone else. Of course, there are fitness professionals that live in the world of exercise for the better part of the day, but there are plenty of doctors, lawyers, school teachers, construction workers, retail clerks, and small business owners that live a healthy lifestyle too. They have kids, they have jobs, they have commitments – they are busy. They just choose to make the right choices in a small fraction of their day, and it leads them to being physically fit.

"Time management is not a peripheral activity or skill. It is the core skill upon which everything else in life depends." – Brian Tracy

Being efficient with time is essential to create changes in lifestyle and make exercise a part of a routine. Time is perhaps our most valuable asset during our existence on Earth. We can get more of just about anything else – money, cars, love, affection – we can get more of all of these things. Once time is spent, it is gone, so we have to make the best of it and understand that managing time is one of the key elements to success with anything in life, including fitness and weight loss goals. World-renowned author, speaker, and time management expert Brian Tracy says, "Time management is not a peripheral activity or skill. It is the core skill upon which everything else in life depends." I will touch a little more on how to make good use of your time in later chapters.

The Difficulty of Change and Creating New Habits

Is change easy or difficult? I think it's a little bit of an oxymoron. Change involves simple, difficult actions in our lives. If it wasn't difficult everyone with the desire to change could change fairly quickly. People that want to quit smoking would quit tomorrow. People wouldn't *go on diets*; they would simply start eating better and reap the rewards. People that want to lose weight and start exercise routines in January would continue all year. These things are difficult for a lot of people, but if you think about it, the acts that involve change are not ginormous tasks. It involves the same amount of effort to put lean meat, vegetables, and fresh fruit in your shopping cart as it does to put donuts, cookies, and soda in your shopping cart. It takes the same amount of time to sit on the couch and watch a few TV shows as it does to pop in an exercise video or go to the gym. If our lifestyle is not one that embraces healthy eating and exercise, then we probably will not stick with it. It is not any one particular action involving change that is difficult; it is our own minds believing change is difficult that makes it so. And our beliefs come from influences around us; our friends, our relationships, the books we read, the church we attend, the hobbies we have, the activities we participate in – our lifestyle.

What is it that makes forming a new habit so hard? I have heard a comparison from a motivational speaker that is spot-on. The temperament of humans is much like the way a thermostat controls the temperature in a house. We are set in our ways like a thermostat has a temperature setting. When the temperature is set in our house to 75 degrees, the heating system is constantly working to stay at that temperature. As soon as the temperature dips slightly it automatically works to get back to the set temperature. We are the same way. We are set in our habits, our lifestyle. As soon as we stray from our habits (what we have *set* ourselves to), we seem to find a way to return back to where we started. Breaking old habits and starting new ones means giving ourselves a new set point so we can begin to live the way we want to live.

I have read in various sources that it takes 21 days to make something a habit. I have seen other studies that dispute this. One particular study found that it takes anywhere from 18 to 254 days to form a habit[1]! There are so many variables involved with making something automatic in one's life. Passion, personality, outside influence, and degree of difficulty can all play a role in making or breaking habits. When it comes to fitness my experience tells me that habits are things that take time to establish. If you are a person that is 30 years old who is a former high school athlete and exercises sporadically, it may only take a month or two to make exercise a habit and a part of your lifestyle. If you are in your 30's and the last time you exercised was in P.E. class in the fifth grade, it may take a little longer to make exercise feel comfortable and become a habit.

Creating an Environment for Lifestyle Change

When looking at creating a lifestyle which allows for fitness to become a regular part of your life we need to look at creating an environment around you that will help you succeed. Below are several key points that can help in creating a lifestyle that involves fitness.

1. Priorities

Our priorities can tell us a lot about our lifestyle. Do you consider fitness to be a big priority in your life? And, if not, do you want fitness to become a priority in your life? If the answer is yes, and if you're reading this book I would assume that it is, then I would assume that you allot a certain amount of time in your life to health and fitness. One big indicator of this is evaluating how you spend.

As a former representative for a direct sales fitness company that sells workout DVDs I have encountered many excuses of why people "can't" exercise. A statement that I have encountered more than once goes a little something like this:

"I can't afford to pay for a fitness program" - sent from my iPad®

Okay, I don't have a problem with tablets, wireless devices, video games, and other modern technological devices (I use them myself). Just remember the question: Do you consider fitness to be a big priority in your life? If you were to rank the most important things in your life, where would "health" rank. I would hope that it would rank somewhere in the top 5. Now, where does technology, video games, television,

We can't get more time, but we can choose how we spend our time.

movies, watching sports, or going to the bar for a few beers rank on your list of the most important things in life? How much money do you spend on health and fitness? How much do you spend on other things? Does your spending reflect your priorities?

Money is not the only thing that can be spent; we also spend time. I don't know of very many people that couldn't use more time in a day, but for as long as we are alive on Earth we are stuck with the twenty-four-hour day. We can't get more time, but we can choose how we spend our time. Thinking of technology again, understand that it takes time to play on a tablet, update and upload to Facebook and Twitter, play a video game, etc. When on Twitter I have encountered tweets that go something like this:

"I want to start exercising, but just don't have the time."

Now, that sounds like a really busy person, right? Surely that person is so busy that he squeezed a tweet into his busy schedule and we are unlikely to see another tweet update for another few weeks from him. Wrong. He continues to tweet, over and over, using up time that could be spent exercising. The same thing applies to other activities. It takes time to go out for a drink, go to the movies, watch TV, play a video game, and read the newspaper. It also takes time to exercise. It takes time to work on your health. Again, what are your priorities? If health ranks above technology and happy hour on your list of priorities, does the amount of time you spend on those things reflect what you value the most?

People that are healthy and in good physical condition do not have more time in a day than anyone else. Fit people are not taking out second mortgages on their homes to afford the latest and greatest fitness gear either. Those who are living a lifestyle that includes regular fitness activities choose to spend a fraction of their income on fitness, and a fraction of their time on fitness-related things. Most of the day is spent working, sleeping, eating, taking care of the kids, and driving to and from work just like anyone else. We all have rent or mortgages, utility bills, groceries to buy, and cars that need gas like anyone else. Those that are fit just choose to spend a portion of their time and money on health. Health and fitness is a priority, and spending reflects it.

Being healthy and physically fit does not mean completely giving up technology and entertainment either. If you are at a point in your life where you feel it is difficult to find time and energy to exercise, I can assure you that if you make it a priority you will see the rewards. If you take the time to work out and sweat a little each day, you might actually find that you have more energy to accomplish other tasks in your life. The more energy you have, the more efficient you will become. There will still be time for entertainment – I promise.

Good health might be something you need to spend a little on. It might cost you a little bit of money and a little bit of time. Do not negate this fact. When it comes to certain things being costly, I think Zig Ziglar said it best: "You don't pay the price for good health - you pay the price for poor health. You enjoy the price of good health. You don't pay the price for success – you pay the price for failure. You enjoy the benefits of success."

2. Books, Magazines, Internet, and Other Media Sources

Do you read books? Have any magazine subscriptions? What about surfing the internet? What sorts of things do you read, watch, and listen to? If sticking with a fitness routine is important to you, then I would hope you are spending some of your time with health and fitness-related material. Staying plugged-in with fitness media resources can have a great influence on you and keep you motivated for a life-long commitment to your health.

If you are someone that enjoys reading books, why not learn something new that can help you in your fitness journey? I am not suggesting that you clear out your library of novels and fill it with nothing but books related to dieting, exercise, sports, and biographies of Olympians. On the other hand, if you

"You don't pay the price for good health - you pay the price for poor health. You enjoy the price of good health. . You don't pay the price for success – you pay the price for failure. You enjoy the benefits of success."
–Zig Ziglar

read a dozen books (or more) each year, having a few that can inspire, motivate, and help you reach your goals would be a great investment.

The same goes for magazines. Gossip, fashion, and sports magazines may be fun to read while you are relaxing, but do any publications of those varieties provide value to you? Think again about your goals. Reading about the latest trends in Hollywood probably has nothing to do with the top 100 goals that you have, let alone the ones that really matter. On the contrary, picking up a fitness or wellness magazine might give you some ideas that can greatly benefit your life. You might find a motivating article that inspires you to keep going with your workout routine. You could find a suggestion that helps you with a particular exercise you have been struggling with. Or, you might find a delicious recipe that you really enjoy and make it a part of your lifestyle of healthy eating.

Most of us spend a lot of time on the Internet, including this author. Surfing the web can bring endless hours of time-wasting activities; or it can bring some motivating, valuable, and inspiring information. When used the right way, the Internet can be a useful tool in your health-minded way of life. Of course there are many articles, blogs, online magazines, and such that provide information that is valuable, just the same as the in-print versions mentioned earlier. But there are also quite a bit of online sites that provide much more than straight information. They provide *interaction* as well.

Who do you like and who do you follow? Most people these days use Facebook, Twitter, or a combination of the two (among other social media sites). If you are one of the hundreds of millions of people using social media to interact with the rest of the world, you can use this to your advantage as well.

On Facebook there are more than just pictures of friends and random comments from co-workers. With Facebook's "like" feature, we can actually join communities of people with the same interests as us. Some pages are more interactive than others, but if you find the right page you can get both information and interaction. This is one reason why I love social media and use it daily. Say you are reading an article about the benefits of running in a printed magazine – you might get some good information. But what if you read that same article from a post you saw on that magazine's Facebook page? You can now leave a comment about that article, or even ask a question: "I really enjoyed that article, but I get knee pain sometimes when I run. Anybody else get this?" Often within minutes, or at least within the day, you have several responses from other people offering advice, encouragement, and further reading suggestions. You now have both information and interaction. Interacting with other like-minded and enthused people can have a big effect on sticking with your fitness goals.

With Twitter it is a little less intimate. I have often heard Facebook being compared to a conversation that happens in your living room, whereas Twitter is more like a conversation you have at a cocktail party. A cool thing about Twitter is it is like being at a cocktail party with anyone you want to invite, from people like you to famous athletes. In my own experiences I have had conversations with celebrity fitness trainers, best-selling authors, CEOs of world-renowned companies, athletes, and more. I have also had the pleasure of meeting fellow local trainers, people looking for answers to their fitness questions, and people that have been inspired by a piece of information that I provided. Twitter is a fun place to interact with people in the community of health and fitness, and you never know whom you will run into and have a short online conversation with.

Social media sites have highly interactive communities, but it doesn't stop there. On the web there are several great fitness blogs and fitness websites that provide great information and interaction as well. You can track weight loss, track calorie intake, get support, and more. You can have diet and exercise questions answered at a number of popular websites as well. Take advantage of these things. If you spend time on the Internet, use some of that time to help you stay engaged with your fitness and health goals.

3. Friends, Family, and Associations

The people that are around us have a big influence on our actions, maybe more than we realize. We tend to live a similar lifestyle as our closest friends; we do similar activities, have similar interests, and have similar habits. Some people have said we tend to be the average of the five people we spend the most time with. We have similar bank accounts, eat at similar restaurants, have similar health, and even talk similar. I believe the same holds true for fitness.

Having some associations with people that are fitness-minded can have a huge effect on your own success in getting fit and staying fit. These relationships can prove to have a positive effect with motivation, encouragement, and feedback when beginning an active lifestyle or living an ongoing one. These relationships can be new friends you meet at the gym, online friends, people you meet at local clubs (running or cycling groups, for example), a personal trainer, a coach, or anyone that lives the active lifestyle that you envision for yourself.

Why is it so important to have these associations? Imagine that you start working out in January. You start off really good with exercising 5 days each week – something you have not done in years. You're feeling good, you've lost some weight, and you have even received some compliments from co-workers about how good you look. Then, mid-February, some of life's events happen. You get sick, you work some unexpected overtime, your car breaks down, or whatever the case may be. So, you miss a week of going to the gym. Then you get a text message from someone you have been working out with at the gym: "Hey, haven't seen you all week. Everything OK?"

You text back: "Yeah. Rough week. I'll be back on Monday."

"See you Monday!"

You then go online and browse Facebook noticing that one of your new friends you met on a fitness page shared a link, "5 Moves that Will Get Your Abs on Fire". You read the article and think, "Maybe I'll try some of those tomorrow." You hit the gym again on Monday and get right back at it. Heck, the week off might have done you some good as you notice a little improvement with your exercise routine. One minor setback; you are up 2 pounds from last week. No big deal though, you're still down 9 pounds since the New Year and you figure you'll tighten up the diet a bit this week and really hit it hard at the gym. You're on track to continue with your fitness goals despite the off-week. The next day your abs are sore from those new moves you learned. And bonus! Those two extra pounds came right back off. Maybe you were retaining water earlier – or at least that was your workout partner's theory. Either way, you feel good and want to get back at it again Tuesday night.

Now imagine that same scenario, only you haven't made any effort to make associations with active people and allow positive influences in your life. You take a week off from working out due to the misfortunes of the week. You're contemplating hitting the gym again on Monday. You get off work on Monday afternoon, tired, still with the gym in the back of your mind, when you get a phone call. "Hey, a few of us are going out for some drinks and pizza. You should come with us!" You think to yourself; *I already missed a week of working out. What's one more day?* "Sure, I'll see you at 6." You go home and flip on the TV and notice your favorite movie comes on at 9:00. Perfect. A couple of beers and pizza with friends, then maybe a couple more drinks at home while you watch a movie. Next morning, armed with a slight headache, you step on the scale. Up 5 pounds! *What?* (More than likely you're bloated from salty food and alcohol, but are unaware of it). You start to wonder if the effort of exercise is even worth it and wonder if you should go to the gym Tuesday night, or just take it easy.

I am not suggesting that you go ditch all of your current friends and go surround yourself with bodybuilders, marathon runners, and tri-athletes to accomplish your fitness goals. But having positive influences in your life through associations can have a major impact on your success, so you might have to make some sacrifices. It will mean there is less time for watching football, watching "reality" TV, going to the bar, and hanging out with people associated with these activities. In most cases, this does not mean cutting ties with people. It means spending a little less time with certain people that are less active and have unhealthy habits, and spending a little more time with people that can help you toward your goals. Now, if your 5 closest friends are alcoholics, drug users, obese, and sedentary, then yes, you may need to cut ties with those people. But for most of us, making new associations means having a few more friends more closely-related to the healthy lifestyle we want to live. Your current friends and associations might even have similar goals of living healthy and exercising more, and they may want to join you in your new running club, fitness class, workout program, or other activity that you are involved with.

A Personal Reflection of Friends, Family, and Associations

One thing that I have learned from my personal life, as well as the conversations and feedback I have received from several clients, is that friends and family might not always be on board with healthy eating and living an active lifestyle. Even though you are doing something positive and productive, others might not see it that way, or are not ready to join you yet. The people around you might not even be supportive of your fitness endeavors. One thing to keep in mind is that currently most people do not live healthy and active lives. As of the writing of this book, nearly 70% of Americans are overweight or obese. It is essentially "normal" to be unhealthy, not eat right, and to be inactive. By eating healthy foods, exercising often, and living a healthy lifestyle, you are doing something out of the ordinary for most people. Regular healthy living is uncomfortable for a lot of people, and maybe even yourself. You might feel negativity from friends, brothers and sisters, extended family members, or even your spouse. Be prepared for this, but don't let it get you down. Most times, unsupportive friends and family are not trying to deliberately sabotage your health goals. People are resistant to change. So your new fitness habits which you are building might meet some resistance. The best thing you can do is keep other positive influences around you. When staying positive, friends and family may eventually view your new out-of-the-ordinary habits as *extraordinary*, and they may want to join you in your healthy lifestyle down the road.

When I decided to change my unhealthy habits and get back in shape, I was met with some resistance from the people I associated with. I lost over 50 pounds in about a 5 month period and I received many compliments, but I also got some negative feedback. I was told all kinds of things: I lost too much weight (I was not underweight by any standard). I clearly wasn't eating enough (I was eating about 3000 calories per day). I was obsessive with exercise (I worked out for about 1 hour each day). I "needed" to eat something like a cheeseburger and fries (I did, occasionally). I received comments like this and other great pieces of advice from those around me that smoked cigarettes, ate fast food regularly, and lived an otherwise unhealthy lifestyle. In the society we live in, it comes with the territory.

Something else happened after I had gone from fat to fit. The more I talked about what I was doing in a positive manner, the more other people became interested. Soon I had co-workers wanting to exercise more, family members wanting to lose weight, and friends asking me about what they should eat. Positive and proactive influence works.

As you begin to live in a way that is different from people you have been associating with for some time, just remember to stay positive and upbeat. You might need to make some new associations to serve as an influence to the goals most important to you and your health. Don't turn your back on current associations that you have, just lead the way to a healthy lifestyle and don't look back.

4. Hobbies and Activities

Personally I like to exercise and I find enjoyment in lifting weights, doing push-ups, running, and getting sweaty. I consider exercise a hobby in itself. Other people see it as more of a chore; they'll do it because it can make them healthier, but it stops there. People often ask me, "What is the best workout program?" or, "What types of exercises should I be doing to get started?" It depends so much on the individual, but the short answer is: The best exercise routine is the one you enjoy the most and will continue to do.

I believe it is important to have hobbies that general fitness routines can enhance. For instance, if your hobbies include going to the movies, playing video games, reading, doing crossword puzzles, and playing

Sudoku, physical fitness is probably not going to enhance any of those activities very much. On the other hand, if your hobbies include basketball, softball, martial arts, hiking, bike riding, or surfing, then exercising regularly can enhance these activities and improve your performance. Again, we don't need to do the 180 degree flip here and sell our video game consoles or cancel our cable TV service, but having one or two active hobbies in place of sedentary hobbies is a great idea.

Hobbies and activities outside of a regular fitness regimen do not necessarily have to involve competitive team sports or events either. Hiking State Parks or National Parks and enjoying the beautiful outdoor scenery is one way to get moving outside of fitness classes and treadmills. Being involved with youth sports as a coach, assistant coach, or referee can add some enjoyment and activity a few times each week. There's water sports, motorsports, scuba diving, rock climbing, and countless other activities that are enjoyable and allow us to use some of the benefits realized from our fitness routines in health clubs or home gyms.

Competitive sports are also fun to take part in for some people. I have friends that are competitive runners, bodybuilders, martial artists, and more. Some of these people began taking part in these activities in their thirties, forties, fifties, or sixties. Not everyone is training for Olympic gold medals or the UFC championship belt, but training for certain events serves as a great motivational tool for people living an active lifestyle. 5K and 10K running events happen in almost every region of the country giving people an opportunity to compete locally. In recent years, outdoor mud racing events have grown in popularity and seen thousands of participants at regional events. With the increasing interest of mixed martial arts, we have seen different martial arts gyms pop up all over the country along with different fight leagues allowing amateur and up-and-coming fighters to show their skills. More traditionally, there are softball, basketball, and soccer leagues in most major cities across the nation. There are a variety of ways for people of all ages to compete and have fun. Finding these activities and participating in them can serve as a great motivator to stay engaged with fitness.

I have a friend that I met online a couple of years ago; she was in her late thirties/early forties at the time, and overweight. With the use of in-home fitness programs she lost weight and got into great shape. As she became invigorated with her healthy lifestyle, she set a goal of completing a half-marathon. She continued to use her workout videos and began to run, run, and run. Eventually she accomplished her goal of competing in the half-marathon, and has since gone on to become a fitness class instructor. She stayed engaged with her goals and saw them through. And anybody can do this at any age by staying engaged in activities beyond the living room, garage, or local gym.

The hobbies and activities that we occupy our time with are an important part of our lifestyle. If your goal is to live a healthy and active lifestyle, then it is a good idea to have some hobbies that reflect it.

The Power of Influence on Lifestyle

I'm not sure where this quote originated, but I have read it in a number of books: "If you are not getting better, you are getting worse." It's difficult to succeed with negative influences in your life, and not only negative influences, but also an abundance of influences in your life without relevance. For example, spending an hour playing a video game, watching a TV show, or surfing the Internet might not directly have a negative influence on your life. But if those things take away from time that could be used for exercise, then they are irrelevant activities that are negatively affecting your desire to live a lifestyle that includes fitness. The previous content of this chapter is about positive influences helping you get better.

I talk about influence and lifestyle from my own experiences in life too. There have been times in my life when I was living a healthy lifestyle, and also times when I was living an unhealthy lifestyle. During these periods I had mostly positive influences in my life while living healthy, and negative influences when living unhealthy.

As a teenager I loved to work out. I played sports, I went to the gym, and I was very active. I had friends that were active too, and I had one friend that I went to the gym with regularly. We would push each other to lift more weights, do more pull-ups, and train harder. I also would pick up bodybuilding and fitness magazines to read about workout plans, lifting techniques, and read motivational stories from the best in the business. Sure, I had friends that were into partying and goofing off too, and yes, I would occasional stray from my workout plans to indulge in teenage mischief; but for the most part I was consistent with exercising. I had enough positive influences around me to keep at it and stay in great shape. As I got older, I eventually moved away from the city in Southern California that I grew up in. My construction job transferred me to a project in Las Vegas. I didn't know anyone in Nevada, but I continued my habit of working out 4 or 5 days each week. Soon I made new friends, and not long after I had moved to the city of casinos, buffets, and twenty-four-hour-a-day taverns, I managed to find a few friends that enjoyed lifting weights as well. I found a partner to go to the gym with me, and had a couple of other friends that I would see at the gym too. Again, enough positive influences to keep with exercising and lifting weights.

Fast forward a couple of years. I am now married with a child on the way and I decide to take a decent paying construction job in Sheboygan, Wisconsin. Now, when I moved to Wisconsin I was not greeted by people saying, "Welcome to Wisconsin. We are going to make you fat." That's not what I was told, that was not my intention, but that *is* what happened. I had a job working twelve hours each day, sometimes seven days a week. The people that I hung out with while living there were not exactly fitness enthusiasts. I spent time away from work with my co-workers – a construction crew whose hobbies included drinking beer, going out to eat, playing cards, and watching football. Without a gym in site, guess what I ended up doing with most of my time? To add fuel to the fire, America's Dairyland has an over-abundance of three things: bratwurst, cheese, and beer – all of which became a steady part of my diet. In just 4 months of living in that environment I gained a lot of weight. I did not have anyone around me living a healthy lifestyle, including myself. The indirect negative influences were all around me. No one was trying to make me gain weight or telling me not to exercise, yet my lifestyle went from healthy to unhealthy as a result of my decisions and the environment I was surrounded with.

Over the next several years, I was doing what a lot of Americans do. I was pledging to exercise periodically throughout the year, and especially in January like a lot of other people. I would do okay sometimes. I would get in shape for a little while, then put weight back on, and repeat. This cycle continued until I finally began to engage with physical activity and surround myself with positive influences again. After traveling to a number of states with my career, my family settled back in Las Vegas again. I began to exercise more frequently than I had in years. I reconnected with an old friend and began working out with him in his garage on weekends. I began to meet some new friends, both in person and online, who were living a fitness-focused life. I began to subscribe to email newsletters from fitness websites and made connections online through message boards with people that were doing the same thing as me; embracing a healthy lifestyle. I attended seminars and group workout sessions with local trainers and celebrity trainers. I was eating better, feeling better, and living better. I was living a healthy lifestyle again, and I had the positive influences around me to help me succeed.

Your Support System Moving Forward

Now that you have read through the past few pages, I have a bit of a confession. Hanging out with people that enjoy exercising, subscribing to good magazines, and being connected to the right websites and social circles are not the first steps in creating a healthy lifestyle. They are not even the things that will cause you to lose weight, gain muscle, tone-up, or accomplish whatever goal it is that you have. The biggest thing that will get you on your way to your health and fitness goals is YOU! You have to be the one the lifts the weights, moves your legs, and resists the candy bars. Your friends, family, books you read, and websites you browse are not going to get you to your goals. You are.

"Why did I read this chapter then?" you say. Because this is a vital concept that most people overlook; I overlooked it myself for years. It is the following chapters that will give you tools to succeed with your fitness goals. We will get into setting goals, following a plan, and tracking your success with fitness – all the things needed to get fit, stay fit, and remain fit. Before we get into those things, I have one guarantee for you in your fitness journey: It will not always work out the way you planned it to be. There will be injuries, emergencies, misfortunes, and other unexpected things happening which can steer you off-course on the path toward your goals. That is where the concepts of this chapter become essential.

If you are creating a healthy lifestyle for yourself while reading and applying the concepts in the proceeding chapters, you will have the support system necessary to get past anything that gets in the way of your fitness goals! Chances are you are not going to find 5 new friends that share a passion for health and fitness and build relationships with those people overnight. You might not be able to think of a hobby that is related to physical fitness off the top of your head, and it might take a bit of searching to find a magazine, website, or newsletter that resonates with you. That said, if you keep these things in mind moving forward, you will be setting yourself up for success and experience a lifestyle change geared toward healthy living.

Apply it to Your Life

1. Do a priority evaluation. What are your top 5 goals, fitness-related or not. How does your spending of time and money reflect those goals?

2. Who do you spend time with? What do you spend time on? What are 3 things you are currently doing that you could do less of? What are 3

things you could do more of?

Tip: Use the worksheets at the end of this book or go to glengoschfitness.com/free for free worksheets

2. SETTING AND ACHIEVING GOALS

Setting goals is an important part of staying engaged with fitness for the long-term, and having a clear vision of your specific goals is of the upmost importance. Lose sight of your goals and you are sure to fail. Stay focused on your goals and the end result, and you will succeed. Most people have an idea in their head of what they want to accomplish, whether it is a certain amount of weight to lose, a certain amount of muscle to gain, or an improvement in health. The want is there, the idea is there, but the vision to make it happen is absent. People fail to write goals down, map goals out, and see their goals through until accomplished. In this chapter we will take a look at how to stay on track with fitness by building a true vision of realistic goals.

Running Toward Your Goal

Imagine the setting of any running race you have ever seen in your life and I can guarantee they all have something in common: They have a starting line and a finish line. It doesn't matter if it is a playground race or a 1500 meter race in the Olympics; all of the participants understand where they are going, what they are doing, how to get there, and they can see exactly where the finish line is. In longer races, the runners understand that they need to pace themselves. They also know where they are at in the race at all times. They know when they are a quarter-of-the-way finished, when they have hit the half-way point, and they know when the end of the race is near by the sight of the finish line up ahead. When a runner has the finish line in his sight, he runs as hard as he can all the way through the mark at the end of the race.

Now imagine if a runner only has an idea in his head of where the finish line of a race is at. He and his competitors are lining up to race on a track with no lanes marked and an organizer of the race tells the participants that, "Somewhere, 1500 meters over there, is the end of the race." Pointing in the distance to an unmarked finish line, he continues, "When I shoot this pistol, just run until you have gone 1500 meters." The runners have no vision of a finish line, let alone a half-way point to let them know where to go. They just run aimlessly with a general idea in their head of where to go relying on their own inclination to know when to stop. Even the most experienced runner would have difficulty knowing exactly where to go and when the race is finished. As silly as this sounds, this is unfortunately how a lot of people head toward their fitness goals. They have an idea in their head of the body they want, the health they want, or other goals they would like to achieve. What they lack is the vision that gets them across the finish line, so to speak.

For years I lacked the vision myself. I would exercise without a schedule and without a plan, and it wasn't until I began to take some simple steps that allowed me to truly see my goals that I was able to follow through with them. I have learned some effective ways of setting fitness goals that have worked for me and worked for thousands of other people. These things can help you see the "finish line" and get you ready for the next "race." They can help you reach your goals.

Identify Your Goal

Identifying your goal is an important step to achieving success with fitness for the long-term. You have to know exactly what it is that you want, and it should be something that is measurable. Vague goals like "be healthier," "lose weight," or "get in shape" all sound good, and there may be a way to measure these things to some degree, but the generality of these goals sets a mediocre tone that often leads to goals being unaccomplished. Goals like, "I am going to lose 20 pounds before my wedding so I look great in my dress," or "I am going to get back to the shape I was in back in high school this summer– able to do 50 push-ups, 12 pull-ups, and run a mile under 8 minutes" are goals that can be measured. These are goals that are motivating, challenging, and provide vision. These goals have 3 important components:

The goals have value. They present a desire or need and are therefore valuable to the person.

The goals are measurable and specific. They allow for evaluation and tracking progress.

The goals have a deadline. They create a time frame and a sense of urgency.

A Personal Experience with Finding Value in Fitness

You know what I love about kids? Their brutal honesty when giving an opinion on something. If you ever want an honest opinion on something, find a child age 3 to 5 and ask away. They won't hold anything back.

When my wife was pregnant with my first two children I had a nasty habit: I got pregnant with her – I put on weight. There is one particular moment that I will always remember. It was on a weekend in which I was relaxing in our apartment in Bakersfield, California on a hot summer day. I had my shirt off while sitting around the apartment having a couple of beers. My young, and very observant, daughter looked me over while honing in on my belly and said, "Whoa, Dad, you look like you're pregnant."

"Well," I said, "tell me what you *really* think?"

Unsure of how to respond, her five year old mind went to work and came back with, "I really think I feel bad for you."

As I look back on that day, I chuckle a little, but I also realize what kind of an example I was setting for my daughter and future children to come. One of the things I value about fitness and health today is the influence it has on my kids. I want to set an example of being a fit and active dad, and not only so I don't look pregnant, but because I want them to know what healthy living is. I see value in setting the right example.

Specific and Realistic Goals without Limitations

Having a vision of a specific goal allows you to take the necessary steps to succeed along the way. What is your goal? Do you want to be able to run a marathon? Do you want to lose a certain amount of weight? Maybe you want to get "ripped;" or maybe you want to go from a weight that classifies you as "obese" to a healthy and maintainable weight. There is a broad spectrum of accomplishments to be had in the realm of fitness and you have to decide what exactly it is that you want to achieve. If you want a body worthy enough to grace the cover of a fitness magazine then you will most likely have to work hard, constantly, every day until you reach your goal. If you want to enjoy the benefits of exercise by steadily losing 1 or 2 pounds a week over the course of 6 months, then your plan of attack might be completely different and 3 to 5 days of exercise each week may be sufficient.

When setting goals, it is my belief that people should set realistic goals without limitations. In other words: Don't sell yourself short! You can accomplish anything you want to do! At the same time, know the difference between setting realistic goals and setting unobtainable goals.

> *Don't sell yourself short! You can accomplish anything you want to do!*

I like to play basketball now and then for fun, and I could, if I wanted to, become one of the best players in my community with hard work and diligence. That is an obtainable goal. Difficult, but obtainable. On the other hand, at my height of 5 feet, 8 inches, I would not set a goal to take first place in a slam dunk competition. Could I train for a slam dunk competition? Sure. I could try, but I would be training for a goal a little beyond my reach. Shaquille O'Neal the 7 foot, 1 inch former basketball star can slam dunk basketballs with little effort. He might have had a rough career if he aspired to be a gymnast though.

Basketball analogies aside, amazing things can happen! You can do 99.9% of anything you want to do. There are 3 gentlemen by the names of Rohan Murphy, Dustin Carter, and Bryce Boyer that share the trait of having no legs. They have another thing in common too; each one is a competitive wrestler. It doesn't stop there. I have known people that have gone from being obese to competing in bodybuilding competitions in just a short period of time. I have seen someone with multiple sclerosis get out of a wheelchair after making exercise and healthy nutrition a part of her life. I have seen a man with prosthetic legs compete in the Olympics. I have seen a man by the name of Aaron Fotheringham do a back flip in an extreme sports event – from his wheelchair! There are many stories of people that face adversity far beyond what most of us know and are able to accomplish what they set out to do. There are also people that believe they are too old, too fat, not strong enough, or have some other restriction that prohibits them from doing great things.

So, what is your goal? It might not involve becoming an Olympic athlete, but whatever it is, do not be afraid to aim high. Just don't make it so wild that you set yourself up for disappointment if the goal is not reached. Make your goal specific and something you really want to do. A little challenge can be a good thing too.

Which "Race" are You In?

Back to running analogies: In the world of running there are many types of races. There are long-distance races and there are short-distance races. A runner training for a 100 meter dash is going to take a different approach to training than someone training for an ultra-marathon that is 50 miles long. Two different runners, two different goals. And even in the case of two runners participating in the same event, some runners will train differently than others. My point in all this is that there is not only one way to accomplish one's fitness goals. The nature of the goal itself and the mindset of the person trying to accomplish it are both factors in determining how to reach "the finish line." One's personality can also play a role in how he or she goes about obtaining specific goals.

In achieving goals related to health and fitness, ask yourself if you are a "sprinter" or a "marathon runner." In other words: Are you going after your goals as fast as you can, or are you going after your goals at a steady pace? In either scenario we need to understand that both sprinters and marathon runners do not just run in 1 race. In achieving fitness goals we are not doing something just once and then stopping. We cannot reach our goals, stop working, and expect the results to last; we have to continue with the journey because this is, after all, a lifelong commitment.

I talked about "what to do" for fitness in the introduction of this book and I am not going to get into which specific workouts you should do to get results. It might be one particular type of exercise routine that appeals to you, or it might be a series of different routines. Some people are able to adapt to a healthy lifestyle and make exercise a daily routine for an hour each day, 6 days a week, and are able to do this for most of the year. Other people are able to start off with the 1 hour per day routine, but eventually choose to scale back. And then there are those that start off by pacing themselves with exercising 3 or 4 days per week and are able to continue the steady pace. Some are sprinters and some are marathon runners. Some are multi-talented racers and change up their routine throughout the year, and the variety proves to be an effective motivator to remain on the path of the fitness journey.

Often times there is a problem with "sprinters" in fitness, especially those that have no experience or have been "out of the race" for some time. They run as fast as they can go, push themselves harder than ever before, then end up tiring out. These are people that start with some sort of difficult and/or extreme training regimen. They go all-in by exercising 1 to 2 hours a day, 6 days a week, and do everything but kill themselves in the process (mentally and physically). Eventually they are burnt out and they don't finish the race, they don't see their goals through. I am all for challenging workout routines, and use difficult training programs myself. They work for me and for many other people. But they are not for everyone.

When choosing a fitness routine, I suggest finding one that appeals the most to you. Find something that you will enjoy and something you can see yourself staying with. And it doesn't have to be the same thing all of the time either. You might want to do 2 or 3 months of really challenging routines, then have a month or two of less strenuous exercise, and then go back to training hard again. You might want to work out 6 days a week for 3 months, and then follow a three days per week routine for a few months. Maybe an hour or more each day works great for your schedule right now, but next month 30 minutes a day works better. It is good to have an understanding of what your goals are and how you can achieve them. Do you need to pace yourself? Are you ready to sprint? Which race are you running in? What will be your next race? What is your goal and what is the path you are going to take to get there?

The Power of Seeing Your Goals

"Goals that are not written down are just wishes" – Unknown.

There is a certain power in visualizing your goals and actually physically being able to see them. Imagining what you want to accomplish is great, but having physical imagery that gives you a target – a finish line – is a strong motivator. It helps you to pick up the pace when you slow down; to get up when you're knocked down; to get that 30 minutes of exercise in even if you don't quite feel like it that day. Vivid pictures and words remind us of where we are going and why we want to get there.

In more than one publication, and in several audio recordings, I have heard author and motivational speaker Zig Ziglar talk about how he was able to accomplish his fitness goals. Zig talks about seeing a magazine ad that featured an underwear model with the body that he wished he had. He tore that picture out of the magazine, hung it on his wall, and looked at it every day, all-the-while taking the steps he needed to take in order to get that same body. After a period of focus, determination, and passion to achieve his goal, Mr. Ziglar began to resemble the man from the magazine advertisement.

I'll have to admit, the first time I heard of writing down my goals and hanging them up on a wall or putting up pictures to motivate myself, I thought it was a little strange. Why? Because most people do not do this. But then I realized something: Most people do not see their goals through. When I began to physically visualize my goals by putting them places where I could clearly see them, my goals started to become achievements.

You can do the same thing: write down your fitness-related goals, or write down any goals you may have. Fill up a bulletin board with the things you desire most, whatever they may be. I know someone that hung a picture on his refrigerator of a person with the physique he wanted with a caption that said, "Are you sure you want to eat that?" Make a photo collage of your goals and make it the wallpaper on your computer screen. Be creative! Keep your goals within your sights every day. Read them aloud often. These constant reminders and suggestions can play a huge role in turning thoughts into burning desires; and turning burning desires into achievements.

Put Your Goals in Your Schedule

Short-term goals and long-term goals are both necessary components of goal setting in general, fitness-related or not. Setting short-term goals and putting them into a schedule is a part of the visualization process that allows you to see a "finish line." Scheduling and setting long-term goals is what gets you ready for the next race.

When going after my fitness goals I always like to set goals at least one step ahead of where I am currently at. I know what workout routine I am currently doing, obviously, but I also know what my next routine will be, and I have another one scheduled beyond that. I am also someone that likes to have variety and mix up my routines. Generally I plan my workout schedule 6 months to 1 year ahead of where I am currently at, and I suggest you do the same. Often times we talk about "losing" weight. A problem that a lot of us have with losing weight is that we happen to *find* it again. If we have something scheduled ahead of time to look forward to, then we can continue with a plan to keep the weight off after we have "lost" it.

A year's worth of planning exercise routines might look something like this:

January – Start a boot camp-style fitness program with focus on building muscle.

February – Continue with the same program.

March – Continue and finish the same program.

April – 2 weeks of a recovery period with light to moderate exercise.

Meet with a Personal Trainer. Begin personal training sessions mid-month.

May – Continue to work out with trainer.

June – Continue to work out with trainer. Mid-month: 2 weeks of recovery with light to moderate exercise.

July – Begin to train for "Mud race." Run 3 days per week, do light weightlifting and functional fitness training 3 days per week.

August – Improve running times and continue with the same routine. Participate in mud race at the end of the month.

September – 2 weeks of vacation with hiking and swimming. Begin sports training fitness program with weight training for performance.

October – Continue with same routine.

November – Continue with same routine.

December – Participate in another Mud Race. Recover with 2 weeks of light to moderate exercise between Christmas and New Year's Day.

Another schedule geared for weight loss over the period of 6 months might look something like this:

January – Lose 20 pounds before wedding. Begin 60-day DVD program to lose weight. Exercise 45 minutes per day, 6 days per week.

February – Continue with same program and finish routine.

March – Maintain weight loss with exercise 3 days per week, 45 minutes per day.

April – Wedding month! Exercise 20 minutes per day, 3 days per week up until week of wedding. Relax week of wedding and honeymoon.

May – Begin 60-day exercise plan found online.

June – Continue and finish 60-day program. Plan the next 6 months ahead.

These routines are just a couple of possible scenarios with scheduling workouts, and each one maps out a plan that can be executed in the current month, the next month, and beyond. It creates a vision of goals that will keep you on track to see them through. We want to take our goals from a vision in our minds to something we can physically see. We can do this by scheduling our fitness goals into our daily routines.

Using Scheduling Tools for Exercise

There are several ways to schedule fitness into your daily life, and by scheduling I mean actually writing down or typing out what days you are going to exercise and when you are going to do it. I schedule my workouts in three places; my daily planner, a wall calendar, and an online calendar such as Google Calendar. Every day I can physically see that I have a workout scheduled when I look at the calendar on the wall. I also receive email notifications via Gmail and Google Calendar that remind me of when I am to begin a new routine or phase of my workout schedule. The constant visual reminders keep me engaged and consistent with working out as planned.

I recommend having at least one place where you can write out your schedule for both short-term and long terms goals. This might be a wall calendar, a desk calendar, a daily planner, or something of that nature. If you are someone that makes a list every day, be sure to include your fitness routine on your list. I also recommend having at least one technological tool to plan your exercise schedule. Most of us spend a decent amount of time on our computers or phones, so having a reminder on these devices can be very helpful as well. Technological scheduling might include an online calendar that you view regularly, a website focused on achieving fitness goals, or even setting reminders and alarms on your phone that tell you "It's workout time" or "Begin weightlifting today."

When scheduling time for fitness-related goals ask yourself, "What is my exact goal?" and "How much time am I willing to spend to achieve it?" Once you have these questions clearly defined, you can begin to map out the next 6 months or 1 year on your calendars and lists. You will now have your own personalized schedule that makes fitness a part of your day, a part of your lifestyle, and a part of your future.

Scheduling gives structure to your goals; it gives you something to follow, like a road map. Goals throughout the year are not etched in stone either – they are subject to editing and adjusting. There is not one single path to victory. You might try something and decide that it is not for you then need to adjust your schedule in the coming months. Slight adjustments, detours, and changing lanes are all to be expected when following a schedule that includes your exercise regimen. Just remember to keep your eyes on the destination for the entire journey. As you schedule workouts ahead of time, I suggest using a pencil for writing. Just remember when you erase something on your schedule, it needs to be re-written, not erased and forgotten about. For technological scheduling tools, don't be afraid to edit along the way. Whatever you use to plan your days, weeks, and months ahead, be sure that fitness is a part of that plan.

Setting goals starts with an idea, a thought, a dream. To make these ideas turn to realities they need to be put forth in a way that sets a clear vision. The constant engagement and visualization of your goals will help make them not only possible but also achievable.

Apply it to Your Life

1. Identify your goal. Make it a measurable goal. Put it into print and put it somewhere you will see it every day.

2. How valuable is your goal? How much time are you willing to spend each day to reach your goal? Incorporate your workout time into your daily schedule or to-do list.

3. What is your timetable for your goal? Give yourself a start date and a deadline. Set short-term and long-term goals then schedule dates and reminders to help you reach your goal and beyond. Use printed or electronic calendars to schedule your goals.

3. FOLLOWING A PLAN

In the last chapter we talked about making time for exercise and using tools to make fitness a part of your daily schedule. In this chapter we will talk about making the most of the time you spend on health and fitness. After all, if you are dedicating a decent amount of time toward something, you better make it worth your while.

When someone wants to pursue a career as a doctor, what do they do? They take the necessary steps to get there, they follow a plan. Those that want to be doctors start in high school. They might tell a guidance counselor their goal of entering the medical field, and with the counselor's help they will register for the classes needed in high school to help get them accepted to a good university. They study at a university for years taking classes needed to prepare for the Medical College Admissions Test. After years of preparation to score high on the MCAT, they can take the test and then apply for medical school at a major university. While in medical school they will learn from professionals in the field, and eventually take the United States Medical Licensing Examination before applying for a residency program where they will again learn from professionals while preparing for their career of treating patients.

Now, imagine if someone that aspired to be a doctor went about it this way: First, he reads a couple of magazine articles about treating the common cold. Next he watches a few TV shows such as Scrubs, ER, and House. After that he even reads a few books on modern medicine to get ready for the USMLE test. No need to bother with the traditional way of medical school and learning from experts with years of experience in the field; he's going to become a doctor his way, on his terms. This, of course, is not the way to go about it.

Fortunately you do not need a medical degree or years of education to know how to go about exercising and find a fitness routine that will help you accomplish your goals. It is however a good idea to seek a little bit of knowledge and learn from professionals in the world of fitness to be sure you are taking the correct steps and doing the correct exercises to get the best benefits. A lot of people buy gym memberships or purchase workout equipment for home with little or no experience in fitness. Simply lifting weights, using cardiovascular fitness equipment (treadmills, elliptical machines, etc.), or doing any other physical activity is certainly better than sitting sedentary on the couch, but exercising with a plan and techniques developed by those with expertise in the field of fitness can be much more beneficial. If you are taking the time to do it, take the time to do it right. Learn from those that have the experience and knowhow.

The Power of Seeking Knowledge and Wisdom

Wisdom and knowledge are powerful things. In the Bible it states: "Blessed is the one who finds wisdom, and the one who gains understanding, for the gain from her is better than gain from silver and her profit better than gold." – Proverbs 3:13-14.

Why should you seek the knowledge of professionals? You could try your own way of exercising and burn some calories; or you could learn the ways of interval training and double your calorie burn in the same amount of time (or less). You could lift weights and gain some muscle; or you could follow a routine that tones and shapes your major muscle groups and has you using muscles you didn't even know you had. You could assume you are doing everything correctly; or you could have a trainer working with you, showing you

> *Blessed is the one who finds wisdom, and the one who gains understanding, for the gain from her is better than gain from silver and her profit better than gold.* – Proverbs 3:13-14

how to improve your form and technique for increased benefits and preventing injury. Professionals in the fitness industry understand things like hypertrophy, fast-twitch muscles, slow-twitch muscles, myofascial release and other things you may have not considered when starting an exercise routine. Fitness is not rocket science, and really not all that complicated, but the importance of having a good plan designed by someone with knowledge and experience of fitness training cannot be understated.

Ways to Seek Knowledge in Fitness for Real Results

There are several ways you can seek knowledge and professional advice in your workout routines. Below are several resources that can be used which can be extremely beneficial in achieving your fitness-related goals.

1.Personal Trainers

Hiring a personal trainer can be one of the best investments you make when starting a fitness routine. Personal trainers can tailor a workout to an individual's specific needs by providing one on one training, feedback, and assistance. One advantage of having a personal trainer is you can ask questions as you are going along and get professional advice on training, nutrition, and achieving your specific goals. Many personal trainers also have specialty areas of expertise which can provide people with specialized training techniques.

2. Workout Videos and In-home Programs

In-home fitness programs are great tools that can be used for accomplishing great results with exercise. Often times these video programs are put together by fitness trainers, so you are getting the benefit of efficiency in your exercise routines, similar to routines provided by a personal trainer. Many in-home workout programs offer a variety of workout videos, a schedule to follow, and a nutrition plan that goes with the program.

3. Group Fitness Classes

The group setting of a fitness class can be a high-energy, efficient, motivating way to exercise that is fun for all in attendance. Classes are usually led by someone with experience in fitness that can provide instruction and tips during the course of the routine. Many fitness classes provide total body workouts that push your limits. Watching the instructor and other people in the class can serve as a motivator to exercise a little faster, a little longer, and a little more intense. Inspiration from other people and the physical nature of these workout classes can deliver great results.

4. Online Tools

There are several websites where you can get some great information and tools to help you build a fitness plan. Some sites even offer free workout videos and schedules to get you started with a routine. Some sites offer online support as well, so if you have questions concerning fitness, nutrition, or anything else related, you can get answers fairly quickly. Online tools can also serve as a supplement to your gym routine or in-home workout program.

5. Books

On the book shelves of stores across the nation (or online) you can find workout routines and tips from some of the top trainers in the industry. Several fitness trainers have written books that offer advice related to achieving your fitness goals. By taking the time to read the advice from some of the top trainers in the business, you can learn how to exercise in an efficient manner. One great thing about books is you can get an in-depth perspective of fitness routines.

The Best Fitness Solution for You

What is the best fitness plan? It all depends on the person. There is not one perfect fitness plan that works for every single person on Earth. Different people have different goals, different levels of commitment, different likes and dislikes. I truly believe there is something out there for everyone. I do believe that every fitness program should have the elements of strength training, cardiovascular training, and flexibility. Some routines will have more cardio than strength training, and some will have more muscle building elements than target heart rate elements, but all should have some element of the two along with incorporated stretching and mobility exercises.

I often advise people to pick a fitness routine that appeals to them the most. If having your wisdom teeth pulled without anesthetics sounds like a better time than dancing to hip hop music, you might not want to sign up for dance-based fitness classes at your local gym. On the other hand, if dancing is fun for you, a workout routine that integrates up-beat dance music and exercise might be a dream come true. If taking on a big challenge is something that sounds fun, you might turn to one of the extreme fitness programs available either at a club or in your home via workout DVD programs. Maybe a more balanced total body routine would fit your desires better. I believe that if you enjoy something, you are more likely to stick with it. Even if the routine of exercise is something that is a little uncomfortable, some routines will probably be more appealing than others.

If exercise is new and out of your comfort zone, starting a routine might not be the most fun thing on Earth for you. If that's the case, I would look for a program that focuses on the results that you want to accomplish. Some programs are geared toward muscle gains, some are geared for fat loss, while others have a different aim. Focus on the great results that the exercise routine will bring you rather than the exercise itself. This positive attitude will help you to want to stick with a program no matter what. After you see results and the program becomes a daily ritual you may actually find yourself taking a liking to exercise.

Enjoying the Journey vs. Focusing on the Finish Line or End Result

Isn't it great to do things that we enjoy? Think of how satisfying it is to have a job or career that you like. Stress levels are low, for the most part, and the motivation to go to work each day is beyond the monetary compensation. Exercise can be the same way. If you enjoy what you are

> "Focus on the journey, not the destination" – John C. Maxwell

doing while burning calories and breaking a sweat, the fat loss and improved body composition are and added bonus. On the other hand, if you hate the type of exercise you are doing, it becomes a daily grind that you drag yourself to do so you can collect the paycheck that is your new body. Personally I prefer to enjoy both the work – or workout – and the results that follow.

There is a famous quote on achieving goals from John C. Maxwell that says, "Focus on the journey, not the destination." I couldn't agree more with that statement and it is a good rule to follow. We need to focus on the journey, or what race we are in, as I have been saying. This holds true for the vast majority of things in life that involve reaching a goal, or destination. Here is a little different perspective though, a quote from boxing legend Muhammad Ali: "I hated every minute of training, but I said 'Suffer now, and live the rest of your life as a champion.'" Ah ha! So like anything in life, there are exceptions to the rule. When it comes to exercise I think it is important to enjoy your journey, but what if you hate exercise? *Oh, the sore muscles, the sweat, the time involved – I just don't like it.* If that's the case, then yeah, the journey might not be all that great to begin with. But as things begin to happen; as you step on the scale and see it's down 20 pounds; as you look in the mirror and see your body changing; as the compliments come from people around you, the once rough journey becomes an enjoyable ride.

I started doing yoga several years ago because my wife told me about the benefits that come from doing it. As someone with a fitness background in lifting weights and contact sports, I have to admit that yoga was not the most appealing type of exercise for me. Even so, I was experiencing chronic pain in my back that would make it difficult to get out of bed in the morning. I also had a condition where I would get a discomforting tingling sensation from my elbow to my fingertips which often resulted in my middle two fingers going numb. On days where the pain was really bad I had trouble turning door knobs and sometimes I would have to ask my wife for assistance in opening a jar of pickles. I had heard of people using yoga to help alleviate chronic pain so I gave it a try.

I was horrible at yoga when I first started and did not get very excited about popping in a workout DVD to do 45 minutes of stretching and breathing. I could barely reach my fingers past my knees, let alone touch my toes. When doing spinal twist stretching I would hear the woman on the video say, "As you keep twisting to the right with each breath, you may be able to see the left side of the room," and I'm thinking "Listen Lady, I'm having trouble seeing over my right shoulder, let alone anything on the left!" But, guess what? After a few weeks of doing yoga I got better at it. Some of my symptoms improved. After several months I felt a big reduction in the amount of pain that I had, and because of this I was glad to do yoga routines several days each week. Fast forward to present day and yoga routines are some of my favorite workouts. Even though I am not the best at it and I still struggle a little with flexibility, I work on it and I enjoy the benefits I have received from making yoga a regular practice in my life. Today I am pain-free in my elbows and fingers, and my back pain surfaces only on rare occasions. At one time in my life I could not imagine myself doing yoga; now I can't imagine myself not doing it.

So, when deciding which types of exercises are right for you, find what appeals to you in all areas. Don't be afraid to try new things and step out of your comfort zone, but don't make it so uncomfortable that it becomes a grueling task that you eventually want to quit. Look ahead to the finish line, the end result, the benefits; enjoy the race along the way.

The Second (and Equally Important) Part of a Fitness Plan

We know that planning is a big part of accomplishing fitness goals, but there is another part of the equation that requires a plan and that is nutrition. Nutrition is a key element in achieving the best results from an exercise routine. Just like fitness, your diet requires a plan. Don't just tell yourself, "I am going to eat better." That is just like saying, "I am going to get in shape." Those are vague and foggy goals that will bring diluted results. Instead we need a direct plan to follow just like our friend the doctor planning his education, or you planning your fitness routine by following a guided, proven workout method.

Many of us know the basics of eating right. We know to stay away from sweets, limit alcohol, and eat less processed foods. We should eat lean meats, vegetables, fruits, whole grains, and drink plenty of water – there is no big secret there. Then why do we need a plan? Fortunately, the past few decades have brought us a wealth of knowledge concerning nutrition. We now understand that certain ratios of carbohydrates, proteins, and fats (also called macronutrients) should be consumed when trying to reach a specific desired fitness goal. Just like a marathon runner is going to have a different training regimen than a bodybuilder, the runner will likely eat differently than his muscle-bound counterpart. Most personal trainers can help you with a diet plan (or direct you to the right resources), and most in-home workout programs provide a guide to follow as well. Just like a well-planned fitness routine will bring you the best results, a well-designed nutrition plan also will bring the best results. A lot of the time people assume that if they are putting in a great amount of effort toward fitness that they will accomplish their goals regardless of the types of food they are consuming. Unfortunately, this is not true. I have heard statements similar to, "The path to a great body is 50% exercise and 50% nutrition," or "A great body takes one part fitness, one part diet, and 100% dedication." Both are neat sayings, and I am not sure what the exact required ratio of diet to exercise is to achieve greatness, but I do know that it absolutely takes both elements to make it happen. Neither nutrition nor exercise should be neglected, and both require a plan.

Which Nutrition Plan is the Best?

There are many nutrition plans and theories floating around today. Which diet is best? Should I eat a vegan diet? Low-carb? Paleo? Something else? Proponents of each diet plan will tell you why one is better than the other. Personally, I think that we are all a little different and what works for me might not exactly work for you. I recommend starting out with a plan that coincides with your particular workout routine. For most Americans this means a reduction in refined carbohydrates and an increase in the amount of vegetables we eat. I have seen grain-free plans, meat-free plans, and sugar-free plans, but I have yet to see a veggie-free plan. If you are unsure of a diet plan to follow, you can look to books or online resources to find a plan that suits your needs. Some websites allow you to enter the type of exercise you are doing, your current height and weight, along with other information to determine an eating plan that is right for you. Perhaps the best way to get nutritional advice is to meet with a dietician or nutritionist to understand your specific needs. All of these resources mentioned can be a place to turn to when it comes to nutrition, and it is important to take advantage of these. This way you will know the proper protein/carb/fat ratio for your specific needs and know the proper foods to eat so you can reach the correct macronutrient levels related to your goals. I will discuss diet and nutrition a bit further in Chapter 6.

A well-designed plan for your fitness and nutritional needs is vital to your success. Finding a plan that is closely related to your specific needs is going to provide you with the techniques necessary to achieve maximum results with the time, effort, and money you are affording for your fitness goals. As you venture on your fitness journey you may find one particular plan that fits you perfectly, or you might grow a liking for a few different plans and decide to rotate between those plans throughout the year. The structure that comes with following plans put together by experienced professionals in the fields of fitness and nutrition is going to provide the best outcome for the weight you want to lose, the muscle you want to gain, the body you want, or the level of health you are seeking.

Apply it to Your Life

1. Do you have a fitness plan? Would you benefit best from a trainer, fitness class, in-home fitness program, another routine, or a combination? Whatever the case, be sure you find a well-designed plan that will help you achieve your goals.

2. What is your eating plan? Talk with a trainer, dietician, online consultant, or do your own research to find a plan that compliments your specific fitness routine.

4. TRACKING PROGRESS AND MEASURING SUCCESS

We have talked about setting definitive and measurable goals in previous chapters, and now we are going to get into how we can measure our progress in reaching our goals. This may seem like something pretty cut and dry that does not require much explanation, but there are a few things to keep in mind when keeping track of our goals related to fitness. Most of us use only one tool, or at least use this one tool most of the time when starting a diet and fitness routine: The almighty scale. While the scale can be one way to measure success in your fitness progress, it is a good idea to have a variety of ways to evaluate the change in your physique and health.

A lot of us are concerned with our weight, and for good reason. An overwhelming percentage of the population in the United States is overweight or obese. Many people that start a fitness program have an idea of how much weight they would like to lose or have a desired goal weight in mind. People might want to lose 40 pounds, or get to a desired weight of 120 pounds, for example. Goals like this are good and bad. They are good in the sense that they are measurable goals; but they are bad in the sense that body weight has quite a bit of variables and may not always be a great indicator of progress. For someone that is 100 pounds overweight a scale is a pretty good indicator of success and will be for some time. On the other hand, someone looking to lose 15 pounds might be thrown off by the number he or she sees when looking down at the reading on a scale for several reasons.

Weighing-in on Weight

Have you ever heard that muscle weighs more than fat? It's true. I once heard that Michael Jordan would have been considered "overweight" in his playing days despite having an obviously lean and muscular body. Body weight does not always reflect fat content in the body, yet people have their minds focused on the scale which measures weight. This is one way that a scale can be a problem. I believe that most people are trying to *shed fat*, rather than *lose weight* per se, and for this reason other forms of measurement may be beneficial in tracking progress with fitness goals.

Body weight also has a tendency to fluctuate, and there are a number of causes for this. The food we ate the day before, the amount of sleep we got, the amount of water we consumed, and the amount of water our body is retaining at any given moment can all cause jumps and dips in our weight from day to day, among other variables. In relation to fitness we can see weight change by the level we perspire and the amount of muscle we are building versus burning fat.

When writing this book I tracked my own weight for 21 days to demonstrate how weight can change from day to day. I had a goal written down to lose some weight after gaining a little during the course of a 3 month shoulder injury. These are the results:

21 days of tracking weight loss. SW = Starting weight. +/- symbols indicate loss or gain from SW.

Week 1	Week 2	Week 3
1. SW +0.0	8. SW +0.4	15. SW -1.0
2. SW +0.4	9. SW -0.4	16. SW -2.2
3. SW -0.4	10. SW -1.4	17. SW -3.2
4. SW +0.4	11. SW -2.0	18. SW -2.0
5. SW +1.0	12. SW -1.2	19. SW -4.2
6. SW +0.4	13. SW -1.8	20. SW -4.8
7. SW +0.4	14. SW -1.8	21. SW -4.2

Total weight loss = 4.2 pounds

These fluctuations occurred despite eating a similar amount of food each day, and burning the same amount of calories on average each day. Imagine if I had weighed myself on Day 1 and then again on Day 15. I would have been in my third week and only noticed a 1 pound drop in weight. These little jumps and fluctuations in weight can often deceive us in the amount of actual progress we have made.

Scales are not the Only Measuring Tools

I am not suggesting to never use a scale, but just understand each time you step on one there might be slight changes, and this is to be expected. And if the measurement on the scale seems to be standing still, you might also notice improvements by taking other forms of measurements. Below are some of the tools that can be used to track your progress related to health and fitness.

1. Scale
When using a scale, be sure to weigh yourself at the same time every day. Even if you choose to weigh yourself every 7 days or every 30 days, do it at the same time on those days. I suggest doing this in the morning on an empty stomach. This will provide the least amount of variables in your weight.

2. Body Fat Calipers
These little tools are an inexpensive way to measure fat on your body. The most common place to measure fat is on the waist area to the right side of the belly button. To be sure you are measuring the same spot every time, you can feel for part of your bone on your pelvis. Feel with your right hand along your waistline starting below your belly button and move your hand toward your right hip until you feel a bone that sticks out slightly. Directly above this point, pinch your fat and skin with your left thumb and index finger. Next use your caliper to measure by pinching your flesh just to the right of the fat you are pinching with your left hand. This assures you are measuring the same spot every time to get an accurate reading and measure your progress. I also like to look in the mirror when I am doing this to be sure I am not slouching when taking the reading.

Body fat calipers provide a great form of measurement when tracking fat loss. If you are gaining muscle (weight) in other parts of your body, the fat calipers can indicate where you stand on fat loss.

3. Measuring Tape
Taking tape measurements at various points on your body can also be a great tool to gauge progress with your routine. Places to measure may include around the waist at the belly button line; around the hips at the widest point; around the chest; around the thighs at the widest point; and at the biceps while flexed.

Taking measurements with a tape can be a great indicator of both fat loss and muscle gains. If your scale has remained stagnant for a couple of weeks, but your biceps have gone up a quarter of an inch on each arm while your waist has gone down half an inch, you know you are still making progress. Depending on what your starting weight is, tape measurements can often show more dramatic results than a scale.

4. Before and After Pictures

If you are starting a fitness routine, please, please take a picture of yourself. It does not have to be an underwear or bikini shot, but any picture that shows what your body looks like now can be the best indicator of the progress you are about to make. Taking pictures every 30 days can really bring a dramatic feel to the results you are getting. Having the side-by-side comparison also validates your progress and can be a great eraser of self-doubt. When we look at ourselves in the mirror we often don't see much of a difference. You might have been losing 2 ounces each day on average, and when you look in the mirror all you can do is compare your body to what you looked like yesterday – not much of a difference will be seen there. But when you have a timeline of photos in 30-day increments you can really notice a difference that you might not have seen otherwise.

5. Clothing

A more loose form of measurement (pun intended) is simply feeling how your clothes fit after several months of working out. At the point clothes begin to feel loose around the waist when you are trying to lose fat that is an indication you are moving in the right direction. If gaining some muscle is your goal and your t-shirts begin to feel a little tighter around your arms, you know you have made progress. You might even need to buy new clothes that fit better; another sign your hard work is paying off.

6. Performance-based Results

If you have not exercised in a long time, or just have very little exercise experience, you may start a routine only being able to do 10 push-ups. Maybe you have a hard time keeping up with your fitness class, or maybe your 1-mile run time is 14 minutes. A few months later 10 push-ups might turn to 20. You might be able to push yourself a little farther at that fitness class, and maybe you shave a full 2 minutes off your run time. Fitness is not all looks; having improvements in performance is a great indicator that you are getting in shape.

7. Medical Tests

I'll say it again; fitness is not all about looks. Living a healthy lifestyle will improve your physical appearance, and your internal health too. Before beginning a fitness routine, it is a good idea to have a physical examination and have some blood work done. Blood pressure, cholesterol, blood sugar levels, and nutrient levels in your body are important measurements of your health. Knowing your current medical statistics in these areas when you begin an exercise regimen can be beneficial. If there are any areas of concern your doctor can address those areas with you. Tell your doctor you are beginning a fitness program and nutrition plan to improve your health and ask his or her opinion of when you should have another examination. You can get an opinion based on your current condition. Results of tests in the future can show if you have made improvements in cholesterol levels, for example, or any of the other areas mentioned.

8. Less-tangible (but Equally Important) Results

Besides physical measurements of improvement we can also gauge our success in other ways. Compliments from friends, family, and co-workers provide a sense of accomplishment when you are on your way toward your goals. After steadily exercising for a period of time you will most likely notice you have more energy, feel better, and sleep better at night. Another potential side effect of regular exercise is improved self-esteem and confidence in all areas of life. Results like these may not be measurable in quantity, but they bring a quality element that is immeasurable.

Evaluating Progress with Tangible Measuring Tools

In previous chapters I mentioned the importance of writing down, picturing, and visualizing goals; creating a clear vision. In the same way, we want to be able to see the progress we are making along the way. We need to be able to see the finish line (our goal), but we also need to see the track we are running on (our progress). So, with written down goals we also need written down accounts of the progress we are making. Writing down our progress on paper, or even using a computer program or online service to keep track of our goals is important because it gives us a gauge of our success. If we are setting measurable goals for ourselves, we should after all, measure them.

A journal is a great way to keep track of your statistics related to your body measurements. Updating the journal often can allow you to see where you have made changes in your physique. In my own journal I keep track of certain stats daily, some weekly, and others monthly. Weight is an easy measurement to keep track of daily, while something like progress pictures are better suited for longer intervals. I suggest keeping track of your statistics and writing down all of your stats at least once per month.

Online sites are also a great way to track progress and stats. Some sites offer tools that calculate your lean mass and body fat percentage among other tools that provide additional means of measurement. Just like a handwritten journal, interactive websites can keep track of your basic measurements as well. Be sure to use these sites often, just as you would when writing down your progress in written form.

Another great progress tracker that a lot of people neglect to use is a workout journal or workout sheets. You would use something like this to track the amount of weight you are lifting, amount of repetitions you are doing, or the amount of time you are spending with your workout routine, for example. When lifting weights you might be using 20 pound dumbbells and getting a repetition amount of 10. After a couple of weeks you might want to aim for 12 reps with the same amount of weight, or try to increase the amount of weight you are using to increase your performance and results. You might run on a treadmill and discover you are running at a 10:13 per mile pace. Next week you might try to shave a few seconds off of that time. By writing down what you are doing when you are working out you will have something to measure your improvements related to fitness performance. Tracking progress this way will allow you to get better at your routine. The better you become, the better your results will be.

Keeping in mind that fitness and nutrition go hand in hand, it also is a good idea to keep track of the food you are eating. Exercise for most of us is an optional task. Vital, important, and we have a certain need for it, but it is optional. Eating food, on the other hand, is something that we need to do and something we have done every single day of our lives, except maybe in special situations. Sometimes even though people follow a nutrition plan they tend to slip a little extra something in their mouth here and there. Most times they don't even realize how many extra and unneeded calories are going in their bodies unless it is written down. Having a food journal can be an effective way to keep track of what you are eating and evaluating what you have consumed over a period of time. With this information written down you can look back at what you have eaten over the past few weeks and see if it is in line with your fitness goals. Another way food journals work is they can psychologically prevent you from eating something you shouldn't. It puts a virtual spotlight on what you consume. You might ask yourself, "Do I really want to eat this if I have to write it down and look back at it next week?" Food journals don't necessarily have to be used to keep track of calories either. A simple list of what you eat every day can tell a lot about how clean your diet is and what kind of progress you are making as a result of your eating habits.

Tracking progress with our fitness and nutrition keeps us in line with our goals. It shows us that we are getting closer to the finish line, closer to where we want to be, and where we see ourselves going. If we find that our actions are not quite giving us the results we want, it also gives us a chance to re-evaluate and change our course if needed. Tracking progress is an important part of staying with something longer than a brief period of time. It sets us up for long-term habits. Habits of living healthy, exercising regularly, and continuing on a path that helps us reach our current goals and future aspirations.

Apply it to Your Life

1. Go beyond the scale. Use tools such as body fat calipers to measure progress. Take pictures for comparison. Write down your statistics and check your progress often.

2. Use a food journal to keep track of what you eat. Use a journal or workout sheets to keep track of what you do in terms of exercise.

3. Schedule a physical examination with your doctor/physician. Discuss any issues you may have with your doctor. Let your doctor know you have made a decision to start a fitness routine and you would like to see what improvements you make in your health with diet and exercise.

5. STAYING ON COURSE AND STAYING MOTIVATED

> *"People often say that motivation doesn't last. Well neither does bathing - that's why we recommend it daily."* – Zig Ziglar

Many times people quit fitness routines after a short period of time and many point to lack of motivation as the reason for not continuing with a new routine. It is easy to give up if you are not motivated. The good news is it is also easy to not give up and stay on course if you remain motivated.

Staying motivated and on track with your fitness goals is only as difficult as you let it become, but while you are on the quest of reaching your goals my promise remains: It will not be perfect. There will be things that interfere with your progress. You will have things that get in your way that are beyond your control. You might get sick. You might have an injury. There will be emergencies, flat tires, bad weather, bad traffic, and power outages that you have no control over that may cause you to skip a period of exercising. Things happen. We have to acknowledge these struggles and distractions as a reality so when they do happen we are prepared.

Be Prepared for Interference and Failure

There may also be times when you mess up. You skip a day of working out for some other engagement, or you have a day where you just don't perform to the best of your ability. You are not perfect either. While life is not perfect, and you are not perfect, it is all perfectly okay. Obstacles are a part of life. When something gets in the way on the path to our goals we can choose to turn around and quit, or we can choose to hurdle over them, go around them, or do whatever it takes to make it to the end.

Another thing to realize is that results don't always come perfectly either. Often times the results that come from regular exercise come later than sooner. Sometimes the initial progress we make is not quite as dramatic as we had hoped. Sometimes we see people getting results faster than we are. The reward seems too little for the amount of effort that is put in. Sometimes we see results and we are making progress, and then bam! We gain some weight back that we worked so hard to lose and experience a regression in our results; or we hit a standstill. We second-guess our efforts and wonder, "Is it worth it?"

These negative things will happen. We need to acknowledge these things, but at the same time we should not fixate on them. Results will come with time. You will accomplish your goals. Have faith!

Remember that we are not going to hit the fitness jackpot. Living a lifestyle that includes health and fitness is more like collecting compound interest on an investment. We do things over and over with little initial reward, but over time we reap amazing rewards. I know, compound interest, saving, and planning for the future are not nearly as exciting as hitting the jackpot, winning the lottery, or yelling "Bingo!" But the investment scenario is real. It is something that you can achieve if you follow the right plan. I have yet to meet anyone that did not see the rewards from consistent effort with diet and exercise (if they are strictly following a plan). You just don't hear, "I've been exercising consistently, 5 days a week, and eating nothing but whole foods for 3 years and I just can't lose weight."

I have read a couple of books that paint a picture of what success in life looks like with steady, consistent effort. The path to success in most areas of life involves slow, sometimes barely noticeable progress. As some time passes you might notice slight changes, nothing to get real excited about. But when you keep your eye on the prize and persevere, your efforts compound into great accomplishments.

Success with fitness is sort of the same. Our steady, consistent efforts are what bring us results that last a lifetime. Except when going after our fitness goals we will likely see brief moments of improvement and brief moments of decline in our progress. There will be upswings and downswings. The problem with most people is they quit on one of the downswings. They fail to see the next step, which includes a slight upswing and the step beyond that which includes a huge upswing with a rise to incredible success. Instead they focus and fixate on the fact that they experienced a temporary defeat, and this leads to failure. Many people expect the results that come from exercise to be a nice steady climb; and in the long-run it is. There are just a few bumps along the way.

If we continue to look ahead and have faith that what we are doing will pay its dividends in the end, we will not have to worry about the temporary down-falls we are going to experience along the way. It is important to understand that this is all a part of the process.

On the other side of failure is success.
On the other side of interference is a clear path.
On the other side of messing up is achieving greatness.

Positive and Negative

You can choose to focus on the negative part or the positive part of the process on the way to your health and fitness goals. Most people tend to focus on negative events in their life. It has been shown that negative events create a stronger emotional response than positive or neutral events[2]. Think about it. Men - imagine telling your wife this before you leave for work:

"You look beautiful today. Can't wait to see you when I get home."

Do that for 9 days in a row, and then on the 10th day say this:

"Your look is a little disappointing today. Please fix it before I get home."

You just gave your wife nine great compliments with only one negative remark, so surely the nine positive comments will out-weigh the sole negative remark. You did after all give her positive comments the vast majority of the time. Wrong! The negative event will surely evoke an emotion and thought that will all but erase every positive comment previously stated. Please do not try this at home! Or, do try the first 9 comments, and leave the 10th out!

Now imagine your exercise routine or your weight loss goals, or whatever your goal is. If you work hard at losing weight for several weeks and end up losing 10 pounds, you will probably feel some level of accomplishment. Then say you have a bad week where you gain 3 pounds back. Are you going to focus on your previous weeks of losing weight, or fixate on the small amount of weight you just gained wondering why it happened, second-guessing your plan and your efforts? I think most of us would like to think that we would naturally focus on the positive results and we would be the optimist in the situation, but a lot of the time that is not what happens. The good news is this: We are all capable of training our minds to be positive, no matter what happens.

We can be optimistic in our thinking. We all know the old 'glass is half-full, glass is half-empty' example in comparing positive and negative thinking. A positive view on certain situations can be applied in several real-life examples when both failures and achievements are present.

Even the Best Fail

What do you think of when you hear the name Michael Jordan? Do you think of the man that missed tons of shots in his basketball career? The kid that was cut from his high school basketball team his sophomore year because he wasn't good enough?

"I've missed more than 9000 shots in my career. I've lost almost 300 games. Twenty-six times I've been trusted to take the game-winning shot and missed. I've failed over and over and over again in my life. And that is why I succeed." – Michael Jordan

> "I've failed over and over and over again in my life. And that is why I succeed." – Michael Jordan

Most of us remember Jordan as the greatest basketball player of all-time. We remember his 6 championships, his game-winning shots, and his tongue sticking out as he would dribble around defenders and dunk the ball. We don't remember him for the times he blew a game-winning shot or the other failures that occurred. But looking back we can understand that failure was a part of the process in his greatness. Among Michael Jordan's failures and achievements, we remember him for his achievements; we focus on the positive side.

Most baseball players that have a batting average of .300 or above (hitting a ball 3 out of 10 times) make millions of dollars. They miss the ball the majority of the time and still are considered great by fans and the Major League Baseball owners that pay their salary. We focus on the great things they do, not the 7 times out of 10 that they strike out or get thrown out in the field. We focus on the positive, with failure being a part of the equation.

When you are exercising regularly, tracking your progress often, and criticizing your own accomplishments you probably will have a higher success ratio than a Major League Baseball player. You will probably fail a lot less than the greatest basketball player of all time. More than likely, you are going to see progress the majority of the time, and regression only some of the time. So keep focused on the progress you are making with fitness, not the few shortcomings that happen along the way. Positive thinking and optimism can be a vital component of staying on course.

Is This a lot of Work?

Making fitness a part of your life and accomplishing your related goals is not necessarily a difficult task, nor does it take a lot of work (unless your goal is to climb Mt. Everest or run an ultra-marathon). For a lot of people, tens or even hundreds of millions of people in the United States, it involves change. The difficulty for most people lies in the concept of change, not the task itself.

You might be thinking, "Do I really need to write my goals down, hang up my goals where I can see them, write down my statistics, keep a food journal, make new friends, change my magazine subscriptions, and all this other stuff?" Do most people really do these things? The answer is *some* people do these things. A lot of people don't. But currently over two-thirds of the United States' population is overweight or obese. The people in the overweight/obese category are not doing the things I am presenting in this book; not taking the time to plan; not taking the time to write things down; not making the change to live a healthy lifestyle. And what about the percentage of people that are active, achieving their goals, and living a healthy lifestyle? Do they do all of these things? There are a certain amount of people that have some level of self-motivation and are self-driven to the point that they can go about losing weight and getting in shape without a bunch of assistance, but from my experience this is the exception, not the rule. I believe people need outside influences to stay motivated and stay on course. All people need some level of assistance and coaching, some perhaps more than others.

We All Need Coaching

When a professional athlete begins to play a sport at a young age he or she needs quite a bit of coaching. Athletes need to learn how to keep their eye on the ball, how to throw a ball, how to hit a ball, how to stand, and how to play. They need to learn the rules, how to score points, where out-of-bounds is at, what a penalty is, and what it means to foul. As they learn the ins and outs of the sport they are playing, they continue to have coaches teaching them new techniques and new strategies to improve their game. As they reach the professional level – the top one percent of athletes in the world – they still need a coach. Basketball stars Kobe Bryant and LeBron James still have coaches. Tiger Woods and Phil Mickelson, two of the most recognized names in golf still take advice and coaching from others. Professional basketball players do not need to be taught how to shoot a basketball and score points; they are however continually coached each and every game of the season.

This is kind of how fitness works. If fitness is new to you, or you haven't been working out for some time and you don't have a set habit of exercising regularly, you will need a little extra coaching and a little extra assistance to get started. You should take the steps that I have suggested in this book. A year down the road, after you have accomplished your current goals and made exercise a daily habit, you might not need as much coaching. Maybe you won't need to write every little thing down, maybe your nutrition level is so disciplined that you no longer need a food journal. But people that accomplish their goals are continual learners. They continue to use the necessary tools and take the correct steps to continue with their successful habits.

The road of fitness can be a challenging path, which is a good thing; most of us thrive with a little bit of a challenge. The challenge can be made a lot easier with a little help and guidance along the way. Using the concepts from this book, such as seeking knowledge from various media sources, working with a trainer or coach, having supportive friends and associations, and some of the other action steps I have presented here can make the experience of exercise and achieving fitness-related goals much better than trying to succeed without these things.

How do I Stay Motivated?

How our minds work with motivation is something that has been studied by psychologists for centuries. The word motivation comes from the root word motive. According to Google's online search dictionary, motive is *a reason for doing something, especially one that is hidden or not obvious*. Perhaps if we understand a little about underlying factors in motivation we can better understand how to keep ourselves motivated with our fitness goals.

There are several psychological theories about motivation with some being very detailed and others offering a more broad perspective. In 2006 researchers Piers Steel from the University of Calgary and Cornelius J. Konig from the University of Zurich, experts in the field of goal setting and procrastination, published a paper called Integrating Theories of Motivation. In the paper the researchers found a common driving force in several previously published theories of motivation[3]. The driving force is *value*.

Value plays a major role in motivation, and if you are reading this book my guess is that you have put a pretty high value on your fitness goals. You probably have a certain value placed on fitness and the benefits that are related. Having a great body might be of high-value to you. Living longer may have value to you, so living a healthy life with fitness will provide that value. Whatever the case may be, you have a certain value placed on fitness, or the results that come from fitness and living a healthy lifestyle.

Related to value are our needs. The things we need in life bring us motive; a reason to act. Psychologists have found that we have primary needs such as the need to eat[4]. If we are hungry, we need food – we are motivated to eat. If we are tired, we need sleep. These are examples of our basic primary needs. We also have secondary needs[4]. Recently researchers have focused mainly on three secondary needs[3]. They are as follows:

• Affiliation – the desire for socializing and sharing
• Achievement – the desire to overcome obstacles
• Power – the desire for strength and prestige, especially when affecting our well-being

Think of how fitness relates to those secondary needs. I believe that fitness, or the actions we take toward achieving our fitness goals can fulfill all of our secondary needs on some level. Our desire for achievement can be met by reaching our fitness goal; the goal in itself is a valuable accomplishment and so we are motivated by the task. Our desire for power can be met by the result that comes from fitness. Having a body that we are satisfied with and we can show off at the beach is an example of something that may give us a sense of power and prestige. Our desire for affiliation can be met with clubs we belong to and social circles we are a part of, and these can be fitness-related too. Being a part of a running club, a fitness class, or even an online community that is fitness-oriented can satisfy our need for socializing and sharing.

We all have different levels of value in the areas of affiliation, achievement, and power. Some of us value one area more than another because we all have different personalities. Nonetheless, these are all things that drive us; things that keep us motivated and call us to action.

Hindering Our Goals

What hinders us? There is something that tends to get in the way of our goals, something that causes us to lose sight of our goals. That something is temptation. Temptation is as old as the story of Adam and Eve. It is something that will always be there, and will always have the potential to work against us in achieving our goals. The greater the temptation, the greater the chance it will affect our motivation.

To a certain degree, we have the chance to regulate the amount of temptation in our lives. If we can control the level of temptations that are around us, we can control our ability to remain motivated with our fitness goals. The more our needs are met with things that promote the life we want to live, the more likely we are to succeed.

Here is an example of goals relating to fitness clashing with a controllable variable:

Setting a long-term fitness goal and achieving short-term goals along the way meet my need for achievement.

Socializing with my current friends meets my need for affiliation. I normally watch TV, play poker, and go out for drinks and pizza with my friends.

In this case the need for affiliation counteracts the need for achievement. The two work against each other. Both satisfy a certain need, and both provide gratification on some level. If someone sets out to accomplish a fitness goal, but is constantly tempted by friends that hinder progress, the chance of struggling increases. Subconsciously we may give into temptation and choose to center our lives on the affiliation need rather than the achievement need. The goal is less likely to be achieved this way.

Here is an example of goals relating to fitness enriched with a controllable variable:

Setting a long-term fitness goal and achieving short-term goals along the way meet my need for achievement.

Socializing with my friends after yoga class meets my need for affiliation. Sometimes I go out for a healthy lunch or out to coffee with some friends from class.

In this case the need for achievement and the need for affiliation are congruent. They are working together, both providing gratification and both promoting progress toward the fitness goal. The temptation to do something that hinders progress toward the goal is not there. In this case there is a better chance of achieving the goal by eliminating the temptations that work against the goal.

This is where Chapter 1 comes into play in a big way. We have to surround ourselves with positive influences; uplifting books, informative magazines, useful websites, and associations with people that are going to have a positive effect on us. In order to be healthy we have to be living a healthy lifestyle with healthy surroundings. It would be worth your time to go through and read Chapter 1 again. Be sure you are set up for success. Be sure you have the proper things in place that are going to promote your well-being and keep you on the up-side of the success curve.

> *In order to be healthy we have to be living a healthy lifestyle with healthy surroundings*

There are several key points that I believe to be vital components of staying fit and remaining fit:

Influences – Your associations, media influences (websites, newsletters, magazines, etc.), and activities you are a part of.

Preparation – Setting goals and taking the necessary steps to achieve them. Planning exercise with short-term and long-term goals. Following a program. Placing a value on achieving your goals and affording the time necessary to make them happen. Creating a clear vision of your goals.

Action – Only you have the power to turn your goals into achievements. Reading this book, finding a fitness program, and planning ahead all mean nothing if you do not put them into action.

Evaluation – Tracking your progress and measuring your achievements along the way.

Motivation – Reading uplifting and motivating books while remaining positive when bad things happen. Always having your goal in sight and not letting anything that gets in your way distract you from moving forward and reaching your goal. Understanding that motivation and influence are directly related and affected by one another.

Get Fit, Stay Fit, Remain Fit

Going after goals without a plan to finish and a clear vision is like running a race without a finish line. It is a soccer game without a goal; a football game without an end zone; a baseball game without home plate. Having a clear vision and the right tools is essential.

If you apply the principles from this book and actively pursue your goals, I have no doubt you will reach your destination. You will cross the finish line and be ready for the next race. You will get fit now, stay fit all year, and remain fit for the rest of your life.

Apply it to Your Life

1. Continue to stay focused on your goals. Review your associations and activities in your life. Be sure you are set up to live a fitness lifestyle and have influences in your life that promote and encourage you to accomplish your goals rather than work against you.

2. Find 3 books to keep you motivated. Look for inspiring books and stories to help keep positive and uplifting thoughts in your mind.

Glen Gosch

PART 2: WHAT TO DO

__INTRODUCTION__

The first part of this book had a lot to do with setting goals and making a lifestyle change, both elements that I believe are lacking from most people's fitness routines (or least not emphasized enough). The previous 5 chapters are essentially "how-to" steps in creating a healthy lifestyle and having a mindset that embraces active living.

In this part of the book we will talk more about specific diet and fitness tips. I had mentioned in the first part of the book that we are not really lacking the information that gets us from point A to point B. Sure, the world of fitness is constantly evolving and showing us new techniques, programs, and strategies to become healthy human specimens; but really the same core values have held true for generations. Here is the common factor in every single equation of health:

Nutrition + Activity

That's essentially what most of healthy living consists of. Other factors may include stress levels, mental health, (both of which are improved with consistent exercise) and more. Your life multiplied by (N + A) = your health.

I don't believe that there is any one single way to go about fitness and nutrition. Healthy living is not one-size-fits-all. I do believe there are several varieties to try on for size in this industry, and in this age of information we can shop around for what fits our lifestyle the best.

Personally I have tried many different diets and many different exercise programs. With fitness I have played organized sports, practiced martial arts, been through boot camp-style fitness routines, tried interval training, did a dance routine (once; I'll try almost anything once), and have tried my own routines in gyms. Needless to say, I have tried quite a few things when it comes to exercise.

With nutrition I have been through a buffet table of plans as well. Low-carb, vegan, Paleo-style, grazing, fasting, and several other well-guided plans. When I was younger, and a little less educated on nutrition, I even tried some plans that I look back at as just plain ridiculous now.

If you have ever tried a diet or fitness routine that didn't produce results, one of several things happened. You either followed a plan that didn't work, or (I'll be blunt) you didn't work the plan correctly. In some cases you may have followed a plan that was not the right fit for you. From what we have discussed in previous chapters, and what we are about to discuss in the following chapters, you might realize that you need to find a completely new nutrition plan or exercise routine. But, you may find that maybe you just need to apply a plan you have previously tried a little more efficiently.

So, throughout my years of trial and error, and what later became research, reading, and applied actions, I bring you the next couple of chapters that give a general overview of what is out there in terms of diets and exercise programs.

6. DIET

Before we get into diets, let's first realize what a "diet" is. Most people view a diet as something that is a temporary eating style to lose weight or realize some other benefit (gaining muscle, for instance). A diet is actually just the way any one person eats. In Merriam-Webster's Dictionary, diet is defined as "**a:** food and drink regularly provided or consumed **b:** habitual nourishment **c:** the kind of food prescribed for a special reason **d:** a regimen of eating and drinking sparingly so as to reduce one's weight." I think most of us think of definition "d" when we hear the word diet. This chapter focuses on diet as an all-encompassing way of eating.

In chapter 1 I mentioned the importance of losing the temporary mindset when it comes to fitness and living a lifestyle that includes fitness. The same can be said for healthy eating. We need to go on a lifelong diet, not some sort of reward/punishment system that involves emotional food deprivation followed by spurts of gluttony.

You will not find a magic eating plan in this chapter that says "This is absolutely the way you should eat." I believe there are several great eating plans (diets) available to follow. Which one should you follow? Which diet has been proven to be the most effective for weight loss, maintaining a healthy weight, and reaching an optimum level of health? There isn't just one, there are several.

In my years of researching food and different diet plans I have seen literature, articles, websites, and other media sources that make all sorts of claims:

Don't drink milk

Drink milk
Americans eat too much fat
Americans don't eat enough fat
Eat 5 even-portioned meals
Fast and eat 3 big meals
Carbs are good
Carbs are bad

There is research that supports all of these claims, and research that disputes them. It has been my experience that one can find research to validate almost any diet plan or concept in eating. Try this:

Do an Internet search for "Risks of a high fat diet."

Next, search for "Benefits of a high fat diet."

If you actually do this (or even if you just take my word for it) you will understand that there are conflicting statements for every concept ever dreamt up in eating. You can always search for "Benefits of (insert diet or food here)" and also "Risks of (insert diet or food here)" and you will find exactly what you are looking for to prove or disprove any diet on Earth. Are you confused yet? Stay with me and we'll figure all of this out, I promise.

Now, personally I have an eating style that works for me (I'll share with you later), but who I am I to say, "I eat this way and it works for me, so you should eat this way too. Everyone should eat this way!" Who is anyone to make such a claim; doctors, nutritionists, parents, neighbors, scientists, and bloggers alike? It is my belief that there are several approaches to eating that work and are healthy. I have personally met people that have had success with the following diets and types of eating (many I have tried myself as well):

Paleo
Primal
Vegan
Vegetarian
Flexitarian
Pescetarian
Low-carb
Point system (Weight Watchers)
Counting calories
Not counting calories

Wheat-free
Following the old "Food Pyramid"
Eating a "balanced" diet
And more!

Tips for Finding the "Right" Diet

Essentially all of these diets work. They might not work for everyone; they might not be the *right* diet for everyone. And honestly, while I have my own preferences, I am not going to tell someone that lost 50 pounds with a diet that I don't necessarily agree with that they are on the wrong diet and "My diet is better than yours!" If you are able to maintain a healthy body weight, exercise for at least 30 minutes per day, and take a physical exam that shows you are not deficient in any nutrient level, then I would say you are on the "right" diet, whichever one it may be.

While there are many diets that are beneficial, there are some diets that are just plain bad. Gimmicks that claim to produce to-good-to-be-true results: Magic pills, injections, starvation, and "instant winner" diets produce a false hope of striking it big with weight loss. If a product says "just take this pill and you will get great results", drop it and run! These diets are the ones to avoid.

So how do you decipher if a diet is a good one to follow? I have a secret to help you determine if any diet on this planet is one worthy of your effort, time, and money. This secret is not science and research that backs up a particular diet with piles of reference materials. It does not involve double-blind studies, experiments, and clinical trials to prove a particular diet's effectiveness. It is not a survey, customer satisfaction rating, or taste test to rate an eating plan or type of food. All of those things are great, and perhaps necessary in studying nutrition, but there is one thing that can test every diet available to realize if it is a healthy plan or an illegitimate scheme. Are you ready for it? Here it is: common sense.

Diet Tip #1: Apply the Common Sense Test

You can apply the Common Sense Test to about any diet by saying the principals of the diet out loud. Here are 5 examples. See if you can pick out the good diets from the scams by using the "common sense, anti-jackpot, non-microwave mentality evaluation test" – in other words, say it out loud and see if it seems reasonable.

1. This diet involves eating mainly meat and plants (fruits, vegetables,

nuts, and herbs). Eating whole grains sometimes is okay (or pseudo-grains if you want to be technical), but this diet suggests that you limit grains as there is research that shows an overload of carbohydrates in the form of grains may actually have damaging health effects. This diet is free from processed food, refined sugars, and artificial ingredients in food.

2. This diet involves eating 500 calories per day while taking a female pregnancy hormone for weight loss (for both men and women). If for some reason you plateau and stop losing weight during this plan you can eat 6 apples (nothing else) in a day and this should get things back on track.

3. This diet involves eating mainly vegetables, fruits, nuts, beans, and herbs, while limiting or eliminating animal products. Research has shown that overconsumption of animal fats can have damaging health effects, so this diet eliminates that risk. This diet promotes natural, whole foods and suggests little or no processed foods and refined sugars.

4. This diet involves eating as you wish. Just sprinkle a miracle supplement on whatever you eat, and you will lose weight.

5. This diet involves following the recommendations of major government agencies. It promotes eating a balance of whole grains, meat, fruits, beans, nuts, and vegetables while limiting sweets. Research has shown that eating a balanced diet can have lasting health benefits.

Hopefully you can see that diets 1, 3, and 5 are ones that promote eating real foods and offer some sound reasoning on eating. I also hope that you can see diets 2 and 4 are diets led by people selling a product that exploits anyone that will "try anything" to lose weight, and both miserably fail the Glen Gosch Common Sense Diet Test. Diet number 1 is generic statement of what a "Paleo", low-grain diet involves. Diet number 2 is the hCG diet, which is in my opinion one of the worst things you can do for your body and mind. Look up the term "anorexia" and you will find the eating style this "diet" mimics; as an added bonus you can take the hCG hormone as well. Diet number 3 is a generic summary of many vegan and vegetarian plans. Diet number 4 is another scam that people waste money on. Anything that says "use this pill, use this powder, use this potion and the pounds will melt away" is doing nothing but melting your bank account away. Diet #5 is the most generally accepted style of eating: the Department of Health and Human Services recommendations on eating. This was formerly the Food Pyramid which has since been replaced with the My Plate concept.

In order for an eating plan (or diet) to pass the Common Sense Test, it needs to have several key components:
• Involves eating whole foods as the primary source of calories.
• It must not include starvation methods; eating less than 1200 calories for most women, less than 1500 for most men (unless recommended by a health professional).
• It must be free of, or have only limited amounts of processed food, artificial ingredients, refined sugars, or any other man-made food additives.
• It must be balanced to be sure each macronutrient level is satisfied. In other words, it must have a designed balance of carbohydrates, fat, and protein.
• It must not make outrageous claims and promises with pills, powders, potions, and gizmos as the "magic" ingredient in weight loss and maintaining a healthy weight.

And all of this boils down to one principle: Feed your body real food that it needs. That's it. You don't need to be a doctor, nutritionist, or dietician to figure that out. With a little research and planning you can find a diet that works for you; there are many that pass the Common Sense Test.

Make no mistake; common sense and status quo are not necessarily the same thing. Common sense statements with food are things like "Don't starve yourself," and "Eat whole, real foods instead of junk food," along with "Don't be fooled by product scams." The status quo and conventional wisdom teaches us that we need grains, meat, fruit, vegetables, dairy products, and some fat in our diets. So a vegan eating plan might not follow what the status quo says to eat, but if done correctly it can still apply the common sense element. The same can be said of any diet that is centered on eating healthy whole foods.

Diet Tip #2: Follow a Plan

Throughout this book I have stated the importance of following a plan when it comes to fitness and eating. There are several reasons for this. To eat healthy you don't have to be nutritionist or be a doctor, but it is not a bad idea to follow a plan from one. So if you are pondering trying a low-grain/Paleo-style eating plan, I would not suggest taking advice from your brother's neighbor at the gym who tells you about his all-you-can-eat bacon plan. Eating Paleo (grain-free) means much more than just eating meat and giving up bread, just as eating vegan means more than just skipping the meat counter at the grocery store. Even following the government's suggested guidelines for eating involves a little planning.

The first reason to follow a guided diet plan is to be sure you are getting all of the nutrients that your body needs. Sure, you can calculate your own macronutrient (carb/protein/fat) ratios and be sure that you are getting the correct amounts of micronutrients including calcium, iron, fiber, vitamin C, potassium, etc. (if you are a fitness and diet geek like me, go for it!) Or you could just follow a plan that someone else painstakingly put together that will fuel your body with real wholesome food with all of the vitamin/nutrient hoopla figured out for you.

Another reason to follow a diet plan is that you will most likely get better results with your goals. You can try to guess what to eat for 90 days, thinking you are eating healthy, and then wonder why you are falling short of your expectations with your fitness and health goals. Or you can go into the next 90 days, 365 days, rest of your life knowing that you are eating what you should be eating to reach optimal results by reading a book, buying a service that provides you with a plan, using online tools, meeting with a dietician, or taking advantage of the plethora of diet plans available.

Diet Tip #3: Know What You Want, Do What You Need to Get There

What do you want to accomplish with eating and your fitness regimen? If you want to be able to have a body that looks like an Olympic athlete, you will need to be on a strict plan with precision in your choices of food. If you want to be a bodybuilder, you will need to eat more protein than most people and follow a plan that involves eating a lot of food to allow yourself to gain a lot of muscle mass. And if your goal is to just plain look lean and be healthy, you might be able to satisfy this goal by eating healthy food most of the time with the occasional indulgence in treats or "cheat" meals.

There is really nothing fancy or complicated with this concept. You just have to know where you are going, what you want to achieve, and what you are going to do to get there. A lot of times you can self-evaluate and know exactly what you need to do to lose weight, to a certain degree. You can determine the level of precision that you need in your diet based on your particular wants and needs.

Diet Tip #4: Have Short-term Plans within Long-term Eating Goals

I have mentioned in earlier chapters how as humans we are driven by achievement, challenges, needs, and values. I also mentioned the value of having short-term goals to reach our long-term aspirations when it comes to fitness. With eating we need to adopt habits that last for the long-term, but it is okay to have little challenges and benchmarks in between. So, in certain situations you may actually want to "go on a diet" in the traditional sense. It is okay in my book to set up a temporary plan that helps you toward your weight loss (or other) goal; just remember to keep in mind that "going on" a short-term diet is a part of a long-term process, not something you can do temporarily and then return to bad habits.

How do you do this? It involves a little self-control and breaking the deprivation feeling that is experienced with a lot of diets. Let me explain:

Let's say a person weighs 250 pounds and has a goal of losing 60 pounds to get to a weight of 190 pounds. Common sense would tell us that person is going to need to eat differently and exercise more to reach that goal (not rocket science). The person, let's call him John, currently eats about 3000 calories each day with a diet that consists of processed foods, sugary drinks, fast food – the normal things Americans eat. For John to reach his goal, he finds a diet that suggests he eats around 1500 calories per day; half of what he eats now! What a change! Knowing his health depends on losing weight, John goes for it. He gets going and sees progress, but after a six weeks he finds himself hungry, uncomfortable, and wanting to return to his "regular" eating pattern. Here's where the challenge comes in. If he can go another 6 weeks and finish this temporary diet, he will have the sense of accomplishment, but more than likely the feeling of deprivation will be stronger than ever as well.

If John is not careful, he can jump right back on his 3000 calorie, no activity, fast food, soda, and hot dog diet. Or, he can give himself a break in which he allows for a little more healthy food into his calorie intake while putting his calorie level at 2200-2400 calories. He may even allow for the occasional treat once a week to satisfy his yearning for chocolate or other treats . This is probably more of what John's diet will look like in the long-term. If John knows this practical long-term plan is in his future from day 1, he might be more likely to stay with his 90-day traditional "diet" that involves a little bit of restriction, knowing that he is not on a path of eternal deprivation. After 6 weeks of a higher-calorie, less-restrictive eating plan John is happy with his current weight loss of 30 pounds, but he really wants to get after the next 30 pounds. So he goes on another challenging 90-day plan that involves a little more restriction of calories and food, all the while knowing he can return to a practical long-term eating plan.

This scenario might not quite fit everyone's goals or description of losing weight, but it paints a picture of what a weight-loss eating plan could look like: A realistic long-term goal with a lifestyle of healthy eating coupled with short-term plans that might involve periodically "going on a diet."

Diet Tip #5: Keep an Open Mind

I like Merriam-Webster's definition of a diet as "habitual nourishment", and that is how I view the term. Often times in my writing online I refer to a "vegan *diet*" in which I sometimes receive backlash comments such as, "Vegan is a lifestyle, not a diet!" Or when writing about Paleo-style eating, "Paleo is not a diet; it's a way of life!" Well, hey, I wish more people were as passionate about healthy eating. Even so, I don't think that any one way of eating should create tunnel vision to the point that we can't see, accept, and be open to new possibilities.

I do not believe we need to micromanage every calorie that goes into our bodies. I like this quote from Jesus in the Book of Luke: "Therefore I tell you, do not be anxious about your life, what you will eat, nor about your body, what you will put on. For life is more than food, and the body more than clothing." The conclusion that I draw from this quote is not that we should not be concerned with what we put in our bodies, but more that we should not be worried that if one eats a piece of meat whether or not he or she committed Vegan Sin, so to speak. And the same goes for any diet.

"Life is more than food, and the body more than clothing" – Jesus Christ

Back to knowing what we want (Diet Tip #3). If you are someone that follows (or is thinking of following) a vegetarian diet, ask yourself why. If the reason is to limit the amount of saturated fat in your diet and realize the proposed health benefits related, then would you be open to eating the occasional piece of meat if doing so provided you with an added health benefit (extra protein, vitamin B12, and iron)? Say you follow a Paleo or other low-carb-style diet and your previous life experiences have indicated to you that you perform better athletically when you have a little extra grain in your diet. Are you willing to break the Paleo Constitution and face carbohydrate treason charges by having a few slices of bread in the weeks leading up to a 10 kilometer race you signed up for?

I am not trying to start a debate between diet and eating lifestyles. I am merely saying to keep an open mind in all areas of life, including the food you eat (or don't eat).

Universal Truths in Dieting

I am sorry if you are looking for the definitive diet that trumps all other diets and you are looking for me to point you to all the right foods to eat in this book. I probably could give you my opinion on the matter by expanding this book by about 100 or more pages, but this book is more about habits than "do this exactly and eat this exact food." That said, I think we can take the knowledge discovered in the past several decades and find some commonalities between several of the most popular diet styles in our culture and apply them to our lives. We are blessed in the fact that most of us are able to pick and choose exactly what we want to eat on any given day. Isn't it great to have such options in our free society?

Perhaps one of the most impactful published writings in American history is a pamphlet that was written in 1776 titled "Common Sense". In it, author Thomas Paine writes, "Could the straggling thoughts of individuals be collected, they would frequently form materials for the wise and able men to improve into useful matter." Though this quote was written in relation to American freedom, I believe that the principle can be applied to anything, including what research has shown us about food and health. If we can take the thoughts and principles that are taught universally across any practical

> *"Could the straggling thoughts of individuals be collected, they would frequently form materials for the wise and able men to improve into useful matter." – Thomas Paine*

eating plan and find a common denominator between all of them, we can then have a diet that anyone could agree is practical.

There is a universal truth in every diet that I have ever read about, tried, or heard of. It is a common trait of the Paleo diet (or lifestyle, if you prefer), Primal, Warrior, Vegan, Vegetarian, Flexitarian, Government-suggested, Weight Watchers, and every other eating style that is based off of eating real, whole foods. Here it is: Don't eat junk food. I wish it was more complicated than that so I could tell you that I had this great revelation in nutrition that is sure to be the next break-through success in dieting. Fortunately, it is not that complicated. Just don't eat crap.

Now, of course some vegans might tell us that dairy products qualify as junk food, but for argument sakes I will be referring to junk foods as things universally accepted as bad for you. The following are foods that are considered junk food by most people:

Refined Sugar – Including foods with processed cane sugar, high-fructose corn syrup, anything with the word "syrup", anything with the word "sugar", and cane juice. This includes soda, sugary cereal, candy, desserts, and more. Essentially any food product or drink containing added sugar in any form.

Processed Food – Including deli meat, hot dogs, sausage, some dairy products, hydrogenated oils, shortening, margarine, tofu from heavily processed soy, and more. Essentially any food product altered from its original state with a multitude of ingredients and additives.

Artificial Ingredients – Including food coloring, flavoring such as monosodium glutamate (MSG), preservatives, artificial flavoring, and more. Essentially anything with added color and taste derived from a lab.

And here are some products considered to be "junk food" by many, though some would argue otherwise:

Alcohol – Including beer, wine, spirits, or any malt beverage.

No Calorie Sweeteners – Including aspartame, acceselfame K, sucralose, saccharin, and neotame. Little packets of sweeteners added to drinks that are also present in many foods and drinks labeled as "low-sugar", "light", or "diet".

Caffeine – A drug present in coffee, tea, soda, and energy drinks.

Genetically Modified Organisms (GMOs) – Engineered food that has had its genes mutated. Currently corn and soybeans along with corn and soy products are some of the most widespread GMO products in the country.

There are probably some people that would debate some of the items listed as junk food. What's my take on the above items? They are certainly not items that you need in your diet. Sure, they might be regarded as "safe" or "generally safe" by our government agencies, but still, I've yet to see any publication that reads, "You need these items in your diet." While there might be research that shows having a glass of red wine and a cup of coffee each day may be beneficial, there is certainly no information that I know of telling people that don't drink alcohol or caffeine that they are deficient in those substances. And the same goes for processed food, genetically altered stuff, artificial sweeteners, etc. You don't need them. As for refined sugars, they might make up the single most detrimental food group in our culture today: Junk food. Check out the list below of the most consumed foods in the United States.

Top 20 Sources of Calories for Americans

1. Grain-based desserts (138 kcal)*
2. Yeast breads (129 kcal)**
3. Chicken and chicken mixed dishes (121 kcal)**
4. Soda/energy/sports drinks (114 kcal)*
5. Pizza (98 kcal)**
6. Alcoholic beverages (82 kcal)*
7. Pasta and pasta dishes (81 kcal)
8. Tortillas, burritos, tacos (80 kcal)**
9. Beef and beef mixed dishes (64 kcal)**
10. Dairy desserts (62 kcal)*
11. Potato/corn/other chips (56 kcal)*
12. Burgers (53 kcal)**
13. Reduced fat milk (51 kcal)
14. Regular cheese (49 kcal)
15. Ready-to-eat cereals (49 kcal)**
16. Sausage, franks, bacon, and ribs (49 kcal)**
17. Fried white potatoes (48 kcal)*
18. Candy (47 kcal)*
19. Nuts/seeds and nut/seed mixed dishes (42 kcal)
20. Eggs and egg mixed dishes (39 kcal)
* Junk food
** Possible junk food

Stats taken from the 2010 Dietary Guidelines for Americans issued by the United States Department of Health and Human Services (asterisks mine).

Of the top 20 foods that Americans eat 15 of them are either junk foods or possible junk foods! What I mean by possible junk foods is the following: Take a look at #3 "Chicken and chicken mixed dishes." Now, a grilled chicken breast on top of a bed of leafy greens with mixed raw vegetables and an olive oil salad dressing could fall in that category, but so could chicken nuggets with a side of onion rings; and my bet is that currently most people eat the latter far more often. Same with #15 "Ready-to-eat cereals." Shredded wheat or rice cereal with little or no added sugar are in that category, but so are cereals with marshmallows and high-fructose corn syrup. Again, if I were a betting man, my money would be placed on the ticket that says most are opting for the high-sugar variety.

Okay, so junk food is overabundant in most people's diets, to say the least. And I have yet to see a good diet plan that suggests eating junk food items. "Lose weight with refined sugar" and "Regain your health with processed foods" are oxymoronic statements. If you want to improve your health, lose weight, and fight disease, you *might* want to scale back on meat and saturated fat. You *might* want to scale back on grains and carbs. But, you will *absolutely* need to scale back on (or eliminate) junk food. Once you have done this, following a low-carb, vegan, Paleo, wheat-free, or any other diet is more of an exploration of what your body responds to the best so that your health is fine-tuned to an optimal level. I will not tell you that any one diet is superior to another, but I will tell you that limiting junk food is an important part of remaining fit and healthy for life.

Eliminating Junk Food Step-By-Step

The concept of eliminating junk food from our diets is obviously nothing new. We know that if we drink too much alcohol it can have damaging health effects on the liver. If we eat too much candy it can rot our teeth; no great revelation there. We have been told for years not to eat too many sweets in everything from the old food pyramid taught to us in health class to TV shows to magazine articles, and beyond.

Oh, if we only heeded the advice of our health teachers and media health propaganda outlets maybe our country would not be in the state that it is in now with gargantuan health care costs, epidemic obesity proportions, and type 2 diabetes affecting a stifling portion of the population. I offer the previous statement not to make a joke, but rather to point out that eating healthy is really not as complicated as we can sometimes make it out to be.

Even though we know a lot of food items are bad for us, we habitually throw them down the hatch. We get stuck in our ways and have a hard time giving up things that we are used to doing. We also have a hard time giving up things we are used to eating. Think of it like this: If you are someone (or you know someone) that eats a diet similar to most Americans, that diet involves a lot of grain-based desserts, dairy-based desserts, processed meat, alcohol, soda, coffee, potato chips, etc.

(remember our Top 20 Foods listed earlier in the chapter?). So you eat some or all of these foods and then you decide to "go on a diet". If you follow any good diet I can guarantee that none (or very little) of those items fall within the plan. This is where a lot of people struggle. They try to quit junk food "cold turkey", and when they do so the deprivation feeling is so overwhelming that they return to the bad habits of eating junk.

One of the easiest and best ways I have found to eliminate junk food from the diet is a concept that I learned from celebrity chef Melissa Costello of Karma Chow and author of the Karma Chow Ultimate Cookbook. Her 30-day vegan cleanse is one that involves a step-by-step elimination of foods allowing for a smooth transition away from potentially toxic foods. I have tried this myself, and though I am not a lifelong vegan myself, Melissa's "cleanse" approach to eating opened my eyes to new foods and concepts in eating. This approach reduces the deprivation feeling with getting rid of foods we don't need in our diets.

My goal here is not to provide a step-by-step plan to get you into a particular diet, but to provide an approach that uses this step-by-step elimination of foods that are generally accepted as "bad". This can actually be customized to your own preferences too. If you don't drink alcohol or coffee, then eliminating those from your diet is a little redundant. The main idea is to get the junk out! Here is a practical plan to do that:

Week 1: Eliminate refined sugar – Grain-based desserts such as cookies or cake, soda, dairy desserts, candy, cereal with added sugar, etc. Be sure to check labels of all foods because a lot of unsuspecting foods contain added sugar.

Week 2: Eliminate artificial ingredients and artificial sweeteners – Anything with the words "diet" or "light" in the title which may include aspartame, acceselfame K, sucralose, saccharin, or neotame in the ingredients. Also anything that includes artificial coloring, "Red 40" for example. Also anything that reads "artificially flavored" on the label.

Week 3: Eliminate all other processed foods – After you have eliminated refined sugar and artificial ingredients, a lot of processed foods will already be eliminated. Continue to eliminate processed meat, processed snack foods like chips and crackers, white breads and pastas, hydrogenated oils, and most packaged foods with ingredients you can't pronounce.

Week 4: Eliminate caffeine and alcohol – Any alcoholic or caffeinated beverage.

If you follow these steps, you can be on your way to eating a pretty darn good diet. Beyond this a transition to a more fine-tuned and particular diet can happen. You can start counting calories, adding up points, eating plants instead of animals, eating more animals, eliminating grains, or whatever diet appeals to you the most.

Eating for Life

What about long-term eating once you have eliminated the junk food from your diet? No cookies ever again? Say goodbye to beer and pizza forever? It again goes back to what you want. If you want to look like an underwear model, you probably will want to hold to a strict eating plan. If you want to achieve a lean and healthy physique but you don't have a magazine photo shoot coming up anytime soon and you are not concerned with being totally ripped, you might want to let yourself have a treat once or twice a week. If you have an otherwise healthy diet, the occasional glass of wine, bottle of beer, piece of birthday cake, or plate of nachos is not going to kill you.

Just remember that everything you do and every choice you make counts for something. You can eat to improve your health, or eat to deteriorate it; the choice is yours. As you find out your what to do path in dieting, be sure you are taking the steps that lead you where you want to go. Whichever steps you are taking, remember to always eat whole foods, limit junk food, and steer clear of gimmicks.

7. FITNESS

I've tried several approaches to fitness including routines that focus on specific areas: Strength and weightlifting, yoga, sports-specific, cardio training, and more. I have come to realize that there is more than one way and more than one type of exercise that proves to be efficient for fat loss, muscle building, or whatever the particular goal you have in mind may be. There might be thousands of different exercise routines that will deliver great results. Within this galaxy of weights, kettlebells, treadmills, pull-up bars, fitness classes, and videos are some common-ground concepts that can be factored into any exercise routine. You'll notice these concepts present in about any plan that you follow. In this chapter I will present some tips you can use to incorporate these concepts.

As you think about starting a fitness regimen keep in mind that these tips are only useful if they are in fact put into action. In the first section of this book I touched on motivating factors and value in exercise. The motivation factor needs to be there with you as you embark on your fitness journey. Something that keeps you motivated to keep moving may be more important in the long run than calculating the perfect blend of cardio, resistance training, and flexibility to achieve the perfect fitness blend. That said, there is a benefit of finding a good mix of fitness exercises and concepts that will be effective in achieving your goals.

Just as with dieting, you will find all sorts of scientific theories and research that prove and disprove different types of exercise routines. *Do this exercise, but don't do that one; and when you do this one, don't do too much of it. Oh yeah, and don't do it that way, do it this way.* Here are just a few of some general ideas that I have come across:

Muscle burns fat
Cardio burns fat
Too much cardio, or "Chronic Cardio" as it is sometimes called, can
damage your health
Excessive weight lifting is hard on your body
Stretching is essential prior to exercise in order to prevent injury
Stretching prior to exercise can negatively affect your performance

There are conflicting arguments in fitness just as in dieting. *So, what should I do more of to get the body I want*? Cardio? Weightlifting? Something else? My opinion is this: Doing something is better than doing nothing, and too much of any exercise is better than not enough exercise, and all of that beats the heck out of not exercising at all. In a perfect world you could take all the research available and do a perfect percentage (whatever that is) of cardio, strength training, and mobility within your routine. Honestly that is not a bad idea, but again, if something keeps you motivated to exercise

> *"Nothing great was ever achieved without enthusiasm"*
> *– Ralph Waldo Emerson*

consistently for the long-term and is delivering the results that you want, then stick with it - even if the latest research suggests that you are doing it all wrong. Make no mistake, I am not suggesting that we throw all research and new training techniques out the window (you might remember from chapter 3 that I am a fan of following a plan); I am simply suggesting that sometimes the best research comes from your own trial, error, and results.

Another component of fitness that supports longevity is the fun factor. If you find something that you truly enjoy, then harness it! It's okay to try new things of course, but stick with what keeps you enthused and motivated if you have found such. Ralph Waldo Emerson once said, "Nothing great was ever achieved without enthusiasm."

Okay, okay, but what if you need a place to start? What are some things you can do to get great results and health benefits from a fitness routine? I offer some advice in the next few sections.

3 Components

I believe that there are 3 major important components of any exercise routine, and I believe they should be a part of every routine in one fashion or another. There are certainly other components of exercise, but I think most are related to these 3:

Flexibility
Elevated Heart Rate
Strength

Every decent routine that I have ever followed or come up with on my own has these 3 elements incorporated on some level. Of course a bodybuilding routine will have a lot more of the strength element than a dance routine, and a yoga routine will focus more on flexibility then a powerlifting routine, and so on. Nevertheless, every good program will have some level of each of these components, and I suggest you follow a program that incorporates these elements as well. Even if your goal is focused on running and a lot of cardiovascular activity, you should not neglect the other elements - they will only enhance your performance.

Neglecting to have variety to enhance a fitness regimen reminds me of the current state of the education system in America. Many school districts decided to eliminate or reduce non-academic subjects from the curriculum such as Physical Education, Music, and Art to focus more on subjects related to standardized testing to improve test scores. Seems to make sense: if you want to improve test scores, practice on test-related subjects. Only a peculiar thing happened. With the reduction of P.E., Music, and Art, academic test scores have dropped in America! The same sort of concept can apply to your fitness routine. You want to burn fat? Just do more fat-burning cardio, right? You might actually want to be sure you are working on building some lean muscle with strength exercises – add the *music* and *art* to compliment your standardized routine. Having a varied and dynamic routine that involves the components of elevating your heart rate, improving strength, and improving flexibility can bring you the best results, whatever your goal may be.

Let's take a look at each one of these important basic components of fitness:

Flexibility

Mobility and flexibility as it relates to fitness involves working on the range of motion of the human body. Improving one's flexibility and range of motion can be beneficial to fitness performance, and in preventing injury during physical activity. This can be helpful not only during workout sessions, but also in all areas of life that include any sort of laborious activity. Whether you are preparing for a 10K race or a long day at work or even childbirth, taking the time to work on your flexibility and mobility will only help you in your journey.

I, along with many personal training organizations, professional sports organizations, and many athletes agree that warming up and stretching prior to activity is very important. There are some people that dismiss this as necessary believing that stretching prior to exercise doesn't make a difference in performance. Others argue that some types of stretching are better than others and too much stretching is counterproductive. Jack LaLanne, often regarded as the "Father of Modern Fitness" was quoted as saying, "15 minutes to warm up? Does a lion warm up when he's hungry? 'Uh oh, here comes an antelope. Better warm up.' No! He just goes out there and eats the sucker." While I have the upmost respect for Jack LaLanne and will be forever grateful for his contributions he made to the world of fitness during his time on Earth, I have to disagree. In survival situations I might not need a warm up. If an out of control vehicle was headed in my direction, I wouldn't warm up to get out of the way; however, if I am getting ready to play some basketball or lift some weights, you'll see me getting my body warmed up and stretched out. I suggest you do the same. If you want to take 10 or 15 minutes to do so, go for it.

How long should you stretch before you work out? I think it really depends on what you are doing. 2 minutes might be fine before a short brisk walk or jog; you'll probably want a little more if you are about to start a 2 hour gym session. I try to do at least 5 minutes of stretching and warming up prior to any activity; I'll go a little longer if I am sore from yesterday's workout, and I'll do a little less if I'm short on time. One thing's for sure though: I do not skip my warm up and stretch routine. It makes for a better workout and reduces time with my chiropractor, among other benefits.

I suggest working on flexibility and mobility with a warm up and stretch routine before all physical activity, and a cool down and stretch routine after the activity. In addition to the warm up and cool down sequences I also suggest taking one day a week (more if you would like) to really focus on stretching and increasing mobility. In these longer sessions, stretch and mobility exercises can really get some extra attention allowing for improvements in range of motion with the body's different muscle groups. A stretching routine can be done while watching your favorite TV show, listening to music, watching a movie, listening to a recorded lecture, or whatever your heart desires.

Here is an example of how stretching can be a part of a workout routine and schedule:

Pre-activity Warm-up
I like to do a little bit of jogging in place or light jump roping followed by continual motion exercises such as arm circles, lunging side to side, and squatting (no weights). If you want to get technical, these movements can be both *dynamic* and *active* stretching - terms used to describe the always-moving variety of stretches. It may be beneficial during your warm up to do some *self myofascial release* activity by using a foam roller (a self-massaging device) on sore muscles or muscles that are about to be used in your particular routine. *Static stretching* such as touching your toes or grabbing your foot while you stretch your quadriceps while holding for 20 seconds or longer may be beneficial as well. Static stretching is what most of us think of when think about stretching – the stretch-and hold-technique. Doing static stretches is a good place to start for most people, and then as fitness levels improve incorporating more active and dynamic stretching elements may work well for pre-activity stretching.

During Activity
Perform *ballistic* stretches such as arm circles, swinging your arms, shaking out your legs, or even just walking to stay moving and warm in between sets of a workout. This is sort of an informal, active rest when taking a little break during a workout. In other words, if you need a break, don't just sit down; move around, shake things out, and keep the blood moving throughout your body.

Post-activity Cool-down
This is where I like to take a minute to let my heart rate come down if I am doing any sort of aerobic or cardio routine or shake out any muscles that were worked hard. Once I am comfortable, I slip into a series of stretches focusing especially on those that were used the most during the exercise routine. I like to do more static stretching and foam rolling at the end of my workouts to reduce soreness (hopefully) for the next day.

Stretch Workout
I am a big fan of taking at least one day a week to really "work on" flexibility and mobility. What I mean by this is most of us are probably not thinking, "Gee, I am really going to 'go for it' during my quad stretch after my workout today." We tend to stretch muscles *enough* for pre and post workout sequences. Taking a day to really see how far you can

extend your fingers past your toes to stretch your hamstrings on a "sit and reach" or how far you can squat with good form to the floor can help improve your range of motion and prevent injury or chronic pain in the future. A stretch workout can involve any series of stretches, mobility exercises, and myofascial release (foam rolling) to improve the body's function. I'll occasionally do these workouts while watching TV (if I'm just sitting there anyways, why not stretch for a while?). I also enjoy doing yoga, which can benefit the body in many ways including flexibility and mobility.

Elevated Heart Rate

Many people refer to "doing cardio" as the way we get our heart rate up. Treadmills, elliptical machines, stationary bikes, or doing the real life versions of these - running, skiing, bicycling - are what many consider to be the "cardio" exercises, or exercises that work the heart and lungs. The truth is that there can be several ways to work your cardiovascular and respiratory systems with exercise. I use the term "elevated heart rate" because there are several ways to accomplish a heart rate above your resting metabolic rate (your heart rate during zero activity) in a way that can be beneficial. One way is to reach a steady Target Heart Rate by way of moderate aerobic activity for a particular length of time. Another way is to incorporate interval training - a technique that involves short bursts of high-intensity activity followed by a moderate or lesser rate of activity. Some weight training routines such as circuit training involve lifting weights or using bodyweight resistance in a series of exercises with little or no breaks in between, and this can bring the heart rate up as well. Certain yoga styles will even get your heart going. Each of these activities can be beneficial to the cardiovascular and respiratory systems.

Here is a little more detail of some of the different exercise routines that can get the heart rate and up and blood pumping:

Target Heart Rate Aerobic Exercise
This involves getting your heart rate up and maintaining an elevated heart rate at either a moderate or vigorous pace. According to the Center for Disease Control and Prevention, about 30 minutes of vigorous exercise (running, biking up hills, playing basketball) is about equal to 60 minutes of moderate exercise (brisk walking, biking on flat terrain, light swimming) in terms of benefits to the cardiovascular system and all-around health. To find your Maximum Heart Rate a simple equation is to subtract your age from 220. For a person that is 30 years old, the

Maximum Heart Rate is 190 beats per minute. The Target Heart Rate for purposes of sustained cardio activity can be anywhere from 50% to 85% of the Maximum Heart Rate. Below is a chart that shows the Target Heart Rates for different age groups.

Age	Target HR Zone 50-85%	Average Maximum HR, 100%
20 years	100-170 beats per minute	200 beats per minute
30 years	95-162 beats per minute	190 beats per minute
35 years	93-157 beats per minute	185 beats per minute
40 years	90-153 beats per minute	180 beats per minute
45 years	88-149 beats per minute	175 beats per minute
50 years	85-145 beats per minute	170 beats per minute
55 years	83-140 beats per minute	165 beats per minute
60 years	80-136 beats per minute	160 beats per minute
65 years	78-132 beats per minute	155 beats per minute
70 years	75-128 beats per minute	150 beats per minute

The 2008 Physical Activity Guidelines for Americans, a report issued by the United States Department of Health and Human Services, recommends about 150 minutes or more of moderate aerobic exercise, or about 75 minutes or more of vigorous exercise each week. If these recommendations are followed, they are proven to have a positive effect with losing weight and maintaining a healthy weight. Exercises that can get you to your Target Heart Rate for aerobic activity include running, biking/cycling, swimming, brisk walking, using cardio gym equipment (elliptical machine or treadmill, for example), basketball, tennis, circuit weightlifting, or any other sport or activity that elevates the heart rate to the Target Heart Rate Zone.

Interval Training

This type of training involves periods of vigorous, intense exercise followed by lower intensity exercise or rest. A basic description of interval training is simply go fast, then back off. Different variations of interval training may include High Intensity Interval Training (HIIT), Fartlek Training, and Run/Walk drills, among others. Interval training has become increasingly popular due to the idea that this type of training is said to promote fat loss at a higher rate than moderate-paced activity. Many fitness classes in health clubs all over the world use a form of interval training. It is also popular with coaches training athletes in various sports.

There are several ways to use interval training within a workout routine. One can use timed intervals by doing a short period (20 to 60 seconds) of intense activity followed by a longer period (several minutes) of rest or lower-level activity. A slightly more intense version would be doing an even 1:1 ratio of intense activity followed by lower-level activity, and an even more intense version would be doing several minutes of high-intensity exercises followed by a short period of lower-level activity or rest. Interval training can also be accomplished in terms of distance. For example, sprint for 100 yards, walk for 100 yards, and repeat. A less formal approach can be taken to interval training as well. If you go for a run, sprint for a while, jog for a while, walk for a bit, and continue to go through the different paces during your laps around the track or journey on the trail.

Deciding which style and level is best for you depends largely on your current physical condition and your goals. Personally I am a big fan of interval training and use it regularly in my workout schedule. To me it provides the maximum benefit of a cardio routine. And anyone can do it too - high-intensity is a relative term. A beginner can pick up the pace of a brisk walk for 20 or 30 seconds at a time and work his or her way up. More seasoned athletes and fitness enthusiasts can use interval training as a challenging element to their particular routines.

Circuit Training

Training that elevates the heart rate for a continual period of time by performing a series of resistance exercises with little or no rest in between is circuit training. This type of training can be done using free weights, machines, resistance bands, body weight - any strength building tool.

I had mentioned earlier that the Physical Activity Guidelines for Americans recommends 75 minutes of vigorous aerobic exercise or 150 minutes of moderate aerobic cardiovascular exercise; they also recommend doing strength training exercises at least 2 times per week within this scope. With circuit training you can kill two birds with one stone: work on strength and cardio at the same time. Circuit training might be one of the most efficient ways to exercise for those want an overall fitness routine that builds lean muscle, burns fat, and produces a healthy body inside and out.

There are several ways that circuit training can be applied, but a general rule is to switch between muscle groups with each successive exercise in the circuit. Beyond that, a circuit can involve a total body routine or focus on one area of the body. You might do an upper body circuit one day and a lower body circuit another day, for example. Another way to do it would be to focus on chest, shoulders, and triceps one day; on another workout day focus on back and biceps; for another workout day focus on legs and abs.

A way to do a total body circuit might look like this:
Push-ups (upper body)
Squats (lower body)
Pull-ups (upper body)
Lunges (lower body)
Military Shoulder Press (upper body)
Continue a sequence of working different muscles with different exercises

An upper body routine might look like this:
Push-ups (chest)
Pull-ups (back)
Dips (chest and triceps)
Rows (back)
Continue a sequence of working different muscles with different exercises

Remember, this model applies to circuit training methods. Other weightlifting routines might involve working the same muscle groups with periods of rest in between. Part of the circuit training element of an elevated heart rate comes from the little or no rest between exercises. In this case we should switch between muscle groups or specific muscles to allow specific muscles to rest. So you are giving your chest a break while working your back, for example, but the body is continually moving allowing for heart to pump, muscles to work, sweat to break, and calories to burn.

Really a Target Heart Rate can be achieved by a number of activities. The ones listed above are a few examples. Yoga, Pilates, and martial arts - or even mowing a lawn, digging a ditch, or shoveling concrete - all can be activities that bring the heart rate to an elevated level which is a key component of living a healthy lifestyle. Whatever fitness routine you follow, be sure that reaching an elevated heart rate is a part of the mix.

Strength

What comes to mind when you think of strength workouts? Dudes clanging around weights in the Hulk Section of the gym? Well, it certainly could be that type of workout, but it doesn't have to be. There are several ways we can work on strengthening our bodies. I had mentioned briefly that the Physical Activity Guidelines recommends working on strength at least twice a week - I agree. Strength exercises are beneficial for the obvious reason of building muscle (lean or bulk), but working on strength may also improve joint health, bone health, and overall body stabilization which can improve function and health in many areas of life (work, walking, and performing other sports or fitness activities).

Even with the known benefits of strength training which are taught to us and promoted by government agencies, health teachers in school, fitness magazines, and Internet sites, still many fear strength routines due to misconceptions. "Lifting weights will make me bulky," or "I want to lose weight, not gain weight," are a couple of misguided statements that reflect the way some people view strength training. Training to improve muscle strength is not just for bodybuilders looking to build biceps as big as bowling balls and legs the size of small children. Strength training, which is in no way limited to weightlifting (i.e. push-ups, pull-ups, resistance bands, resistance machines, etc.), is an important part of fitness for men and women of all ages that can fulfill a wide range of goals relating to health and body composition.

Strength training is not just for bodybuilders

To put myths to rest, strength training will not make you bulky – unless you want it to. Someone following a bodybuilding workout plan and eating a very large amount of calories can and will add bulk. On the other hand, someone that uses a combination of strength training exercises 2 or 3 times per week using relatively low-load weights, other resistance equipment, and bodyweight exercises with high repetitions will build strength and muscle tone without massive muscle gains. There are several other ways to go about strength training as well. Different styles of different resistance exercises produce different results. Here are a few basic rules for weight training:

Strength Training for Muscle Tone, Fat Loss, and General Fitness – Exercises may include bodyweight resistance such as push-ups, pull ups, dips, and lunges with free weights, resistance bands, machines, and other equipment. Use low-load resistance with around 12 to 20 repetitions per exercise, on most exercises. Circuit training is a good method for this.

Strength Training For Increased Muscle Size – Exercises may include the use of bodyweight exercises, free weights, resistance bands, machines, and other equipment. Use moderate to heavy load resistance with 6 to12 reps per exercise, on most exercises. The circuit training method can be used for this goal, but a method of performing exercises with brief periods of rest (1 to 2 minutes) in between can be applied as well.

Strength Training for Maximum Strength – Exercises may include bodyweight exercises, resistance bands, machines, and other equipment, but generally free weights are used the majority of the time when lifting to increase maximum strength. Lift heavy loads with anywhere from 1 to 5 reps on most exercises. Generally a brief period of rest is needed between exercises.

Strength Training for Power and Performance – Exercises may include bodyweight exercises, resistance bands, machines, medicine balls, and other equipment. A style of exercise for this goal may include *plyometrics* also known as reactive movements such as jump squats. Speed and explosiveness are elements that may also be brought in here to enhance athletic performance. Sprinting elements are also common for working different muscle fibers used in athletics. Load and repetition count can vary immensely with this style of training – there may be a combination of heavy resistance with low reps and light resistance with high reps.

The previous 4 paragraphs are some general rules for strength training, but there are of course exceptions to the rules. When strength training for muscle size one will probably want to lift relatively heavy loads with 6 to 12 repetitions, but when doing a set of push-ups 6 reps is probably too few. And even with women and men that aren't really looking to bulk up, lifting some heavier weights on certain exercises may be more practical. Other exceptions apply as well – it all depends on your individual goals.

It is important for anyone to incorporate strength training into his or her fitness routine, and the type of training can be tailored to each person's individual needs and goals. Whether you want to lose weight or gain weight - strengthening your muscles, joints, and bones can bring a variety of physical benefits.

Wrapping it Up

So there you have it: Cardio, strength, and flexibility/mobility – the things you need in fitness. Are there other components? Yes. Those with a background in fitness may be reading this and thinking "You missed balance, core strength, hypertrophy specifics, functional fitness, speed, agility, and other important elements of fitness." To this I say, "Read chapter 3." I think everyone should follow a well-designed plan that incorporates specific elements related to one's specific goals. I also know from experience that often people neglect an area of fitness. *"I've been jogging 3 days a week and eating better; why am I not losing weight?"* If you happen to fall into the latter category, this chapter is especially for you. It might be time to pick up a book, contact a personal trainer, subscribe to a fitness magazine, order a set of workout DVDs, or do any or all of the above. Whatever route you chose, be sure to have a dynamic routine that does not neglect any of the basic elements of fitness: elevated heart rate, strength, and flexibility. If you are following a good plan, other more specific elements of fitness will fill themselves in along the way.

It's now time to seek a path, get started, and find your fitness. Try new things, find what works, and stay with it – make adjustments in your course during the journey. Whatever you do, Keep moving.

Special Thanks

First and foremost, thank you God for the blessings bestowed upon me. With you, all things are possible. Thank you Jesus.

Quotes from this book were used with permission from the following:

Quotes from Zig Ziglar were used with permission from the Ziglar company and family. Quotes were accessed from www.ziglar.com. Zig Ziglar was one of the greatest motivational authors and speakers of our time. I continue to read Mr. Ziglar's books and listen to recordings of his seminars. I also continually follow his legacy and the work of his family at Ziglar.

Quotes from John C. Maxwell were used with permission from The John Maxwell company. John C. Maxwell has served as a big influence in my life during recent years. His teachings through books, audio recordings, and articles are so profound and applicable to so many areas of life. Copyright 2013 The John Maxwell Company. Article excerpts were accessed via www.johnmaxwell.com and may not be reprinted or reproduced without written permission from the John Maxwell Company, except for brief quotations in critical reviews or articles.

Quotes from Brian Tracy were used by permission from Brian Tracy International. Brian Tracy is Chairman and CEO of Brian Tracy International, a company specializing in in the training and development of individuals and organizations. Brian's goal is to help people achieve their personal and business goals faster and easier than they ever imagined. He has consulted for more than 1000 companies and addressed more than 5,000,000 people in 5000 talks throughout the U.S., Canada, and 55 other countries worldwide. As a keynote speaker he addresses more than 250,000 people each year. Brian Tracy's books and personal development programs have helped me immensely. For more info about Brian Tracy and his programs, go to www.briantracy.com.

ABOUT THE AUTHOR

Why is the "About the Author" section always in 3rd person?

I am Glen Gosch, thank you for taking the time to read this book – I hope you enjoyed it!

I am a husband and father with an amazing wife and wonderful children, all of whom are my best friends. We have lived in everywhere from Las Vegas, Nevada to Kotlik, Alaska and places in between. Life has been great to us, God has blessed us.

Relating to fitness: I was a young athlete quite a few years ago. I enjoyed playing sports since age 6 and continued into my high school years. Eventually I ended my journey with team sports and found an interest in weightlifting. I made some bad decisions in my later teen years into my early twenties. Bad influences, bad habits, and bad lifestyle – both mind and body. I eventually got back on track and turned things around with by making better lifestyle choices and seeking the help of God. Professionally I am a certified personal trainer and continue to educate myself to help others live a healthy lifestyle.

In the present I try to share things from my past experiences that may help other people. I share positive messages and set a positive example by living a healthy and faith-focused life.

REFERENCES

1. Lally, Phillipa, Cornelia HM Jaarsveld, Henry HW Potts, and Jane Wardle. "How Are Habits Formed: Modelling Habit Formation in the Real World." *European Journal of Social Psychology* 40.6 (2010): 998-1009. *Wiley Online Library*. John Wiley and Sons, Inc, 16 July 2009. Web. 1 Jan. 2013.

2. Taylor, Shelley E. "Asymmetrical Effects of Positive and Negative Events: The Mobilization-Minimization Hypothesis." *Psychological Bulletin* 110.1 (1991): 67-85. *UCLA Social Neuroscience Lab*. University of Califronia, Los Angeles. Web. 1 Jan. 2013.Copyright 1991 by the American Psychological Association, Inc.

3. Steel, Piers, and Cornelius J. Konig. "Integrating Theories of Motivation." *Academy of Management Review* 31.4 (2006): 889-913. *University of Calgary*. Web. 1 Jan. 2013.

4. Cherry, Kendra. "Murray's Theory of Psychogenic Needs." *About.com Psychology*. About.com, n.d. Web. 01 Jan. 2013.

Don't just read about it; do it! Apply it to your life:

Do a priority evaluation. What are your top 5 goals, fitness-related or not. Think: does your spending of time and money reflect those goals?

1.

2.

3.

4.

5.

What things need to change so your spending reflects your goals?

Who do you spend time with? What do you spend time on? What are 3 things you are currently doing that you could do less of? What are 3 things you could do more of?

I need to do these 3 things more:

1.

2.

3.

I need to do less of these things:

1.

2.

3.

How valuable is your goal? How much time are you willing to spend each day to reach your goal? Incorporate your workout time into your daily schedule or to-do list.

Amount of time I will realistically spend on my goal:

What is your timetable for your fitness goal(s)? Give yourself a start date and a deadline. Set short-term and long-term goals then schedule dates and reminders to help you reach your goal and beyond. Use printed or electronic calendars to schedule your goals.

I will begin to work on my goal on this day:

Identify your goal. Make it a measurable goal. Put it into print and put it somewhere you will see it every day.

Example: I will lose 25 pounds before May by exercising 5 times per week and meeting with a personal trainer so I can look good for my vacation!

My specific, valuable, and measurable goal with a deadline is:

Do you have a fitness plan? Would you benefit best from a trainer, fitness class, in-home fitness program, another routine, or a combination? Whatever the case, be sure you find a well-designed plan that will help you achieve your goals.

The next fitness plan that I will follow is:

What is your eating plan? Talk with a trainer, dietician, online consultant, or do your own research to find a plan that compliments your specific fitness routine.

The resource(s) I will use for an eating plan are:

Go beyond the scale. Use tools such as body fat calipers to measure progress. Take pictures for comparison. Write down your statistics and check your progress often.

Use a food journal to keep track of what you eat. Use a journal or workout sheets to keep track of what you do in terms of exercise.

Schedule a physical examination with your doctor/physician. Discuss any issues you may have with your doctor. Let your doctor know you have made a decision to start a fitness routine and you would like to see what improvements you make in your health with diet and exercise.

Checklist:
Body fat calipers
Scale
Tape Measure
Before Pictures
Journal

Exam date with my doctor:

Continue to stay focused on your goals. Review your associations and activities in your life. Be sure you are set up to live a fitness lifestyle and have influences in your life that promote and encourage you to accomplish your goals rather than work against you.

Find 3 books to keep you motivated. Look for inspiring books and stories to help keep positive and uplifting thoughts in your mind.

3 Books I can read are:

1.

2.

3.

Suggested authors:
Zig Ziglar
Jim Rohn
Norman Vincent Peale
John Maxwell
Brian Tracy
Ralph Waldo Emerson

These are a few suggestions to get started and some of my favorites. There are thousands of books available that can change your life. The Bible is another good one.

For more from me, visit:

Blog: glengoschfitness.com

Facebook: facebook.com/glengoschfitness

Twitter: @glengosch

www.ingramcontent.com/pod-product-compliance
Lightning Source LLC
Chambersburg PA
CBHW060513280326
41933CB00014B/2944